What I Wish I knew About Cancer

Marty Wilson & Gary Bertwistle

16
EasyRead Large

RHYW

Copyright Page from the Original Book

First published 2011

Big Sky Publishing Pty Ltd

PO Box 303, Newport, NSW 2106, Australia

Phone: (61 2) 9918 2168
Fax: (61 2) 9918 2396
Email: info@bigskypublishing.com.au
Web: www.bigskypublishing.com.au

Cover design and typesetting: Think Productions

National Library of Australia Cataloguing-in-Publication entry
Author: Wilson, Marty.
Title: What I wish I knew about cancer / Marty Wilson, Gary Bertwistle.
ISBN: 9780987057426 (pbk.)
Subjects: Cancer--Popular works. Cancer--Prevention.
Other Authors/Contributors: Bertwistle, Gary.
Dewey Number: 616.994

"When cancer is first diagnosed, some people start to die almost immediately; others start to live. The choice is yours."

Warrick Try

INTRODUCTION

"So far in life I have been incredibly lucky, I have only had two people close to me die of cancer."

The first was my grandfather, Donny, who let me move in with him when I was having typical teenage battles with my Dad (that were all Dad's fault, of course). Donny had a profound influence on my character and I still wear his wedding band to this day.

The second person I lost to cancer was Danny Francis, a friend from university days. Dan was a gregarious, larger than life character whose death in 2010 proved to me that cancer doesn't care how invincible you think you are, it will still have a damned good crack at you.

When Gary Bertwistle said he thought doing a What I Wish I Knew book on cancer was a good idea I was quietly pleased, when he told me that the Tour de Cure would like to produce the book with me, I was absolutely thrilled.

I'd like to dedicate this book to Donny, Dan, and everyone at the Tour de Cure who are working (and riding) their butts off, doing an absolutely amazing job at having a damned good crack right back at cancer.

Marty

"In 2007 I sat in a coffee shop after a ride with a mate of mine, Geoff Coombes. Over that coffee we had a dream-to do our bit to help find a cure to cancer."

Since that time, the Tour de Cure has raised $4 million dollars in cash contributions towards research, support and prevention of cancer in men, women and children, and in doing so has become Australia's leading cycling foundation.

What I Wish I Knew About Cancer is the next step for us in helping people understand what can be done to prevent cancer. This book has been written specifically to share first hand messages from those who have been at the pointy end of cancer. Survivors, pre-viviors, partners, husbands, wives, children, researchers, doctors and even those closest to our foundation, our Tour riders and support crew. We want to further people's awareness around cancer, and in particular, what we can do to better our chances of never hearing those fateful words 'I'm sorry, you have cancer.'

It has been amazing journey for Geoff and I, and we hope this book takes us one small step closer to a cure.

DANIEL WALTERS

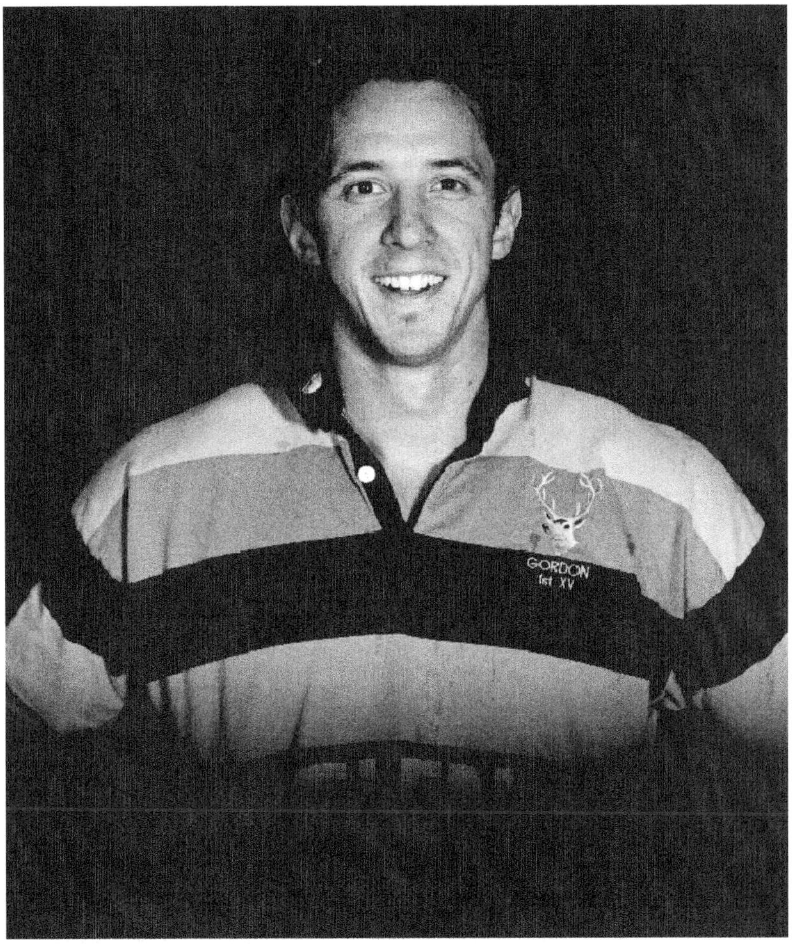

"You wouldn't wish three months of chemo on your worst enemy. It is the most disgusting, barbaric, inhumane way to treat a disease, but it worked, so I'd do it again tomorrow."

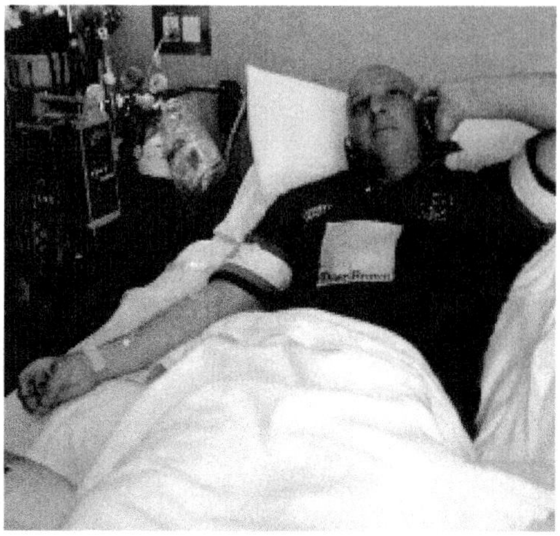

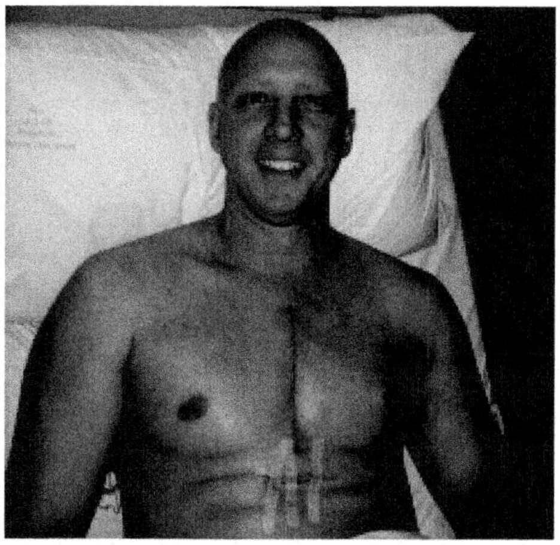

"Control the controllables. Don't worry about what the oncologist is doing; he does it all day every day, so you don't have to be concerned about the type of chemo, what's in the chemo, the dose etc. Just focus on what you can control."

"Every time I was sick I'd picture a little bit of the tumour coming out. Every vomit, a little bit more came out. So the sicker I was, in my mind, the better I was getting."

At the age of 28, having just completed five years of chiropractic study, Daniel Walters started feeling unwell. He was sweating a lot, feeling tired and lethargic, falling into bed at 7 pm each night, and needing to have a two hour sleep each day. After repeated trips to the GP, ultrasounds, a lymph node biopsy and continually being given the all clear, Daniel was sent for a CT scan where they found the cause of his constant exhaustion: a fist sized tumour wrapped around the aorta and superior vena cava near his heart, which was actually a rare and aggressive form of testicular cancer. Now, aged 33, Daniel is in remission and feels blessed to have recently become a father.

"Cancer to me, before I had it, was an old man's disease. It was something you got at the end of your time."

MEL CAIN

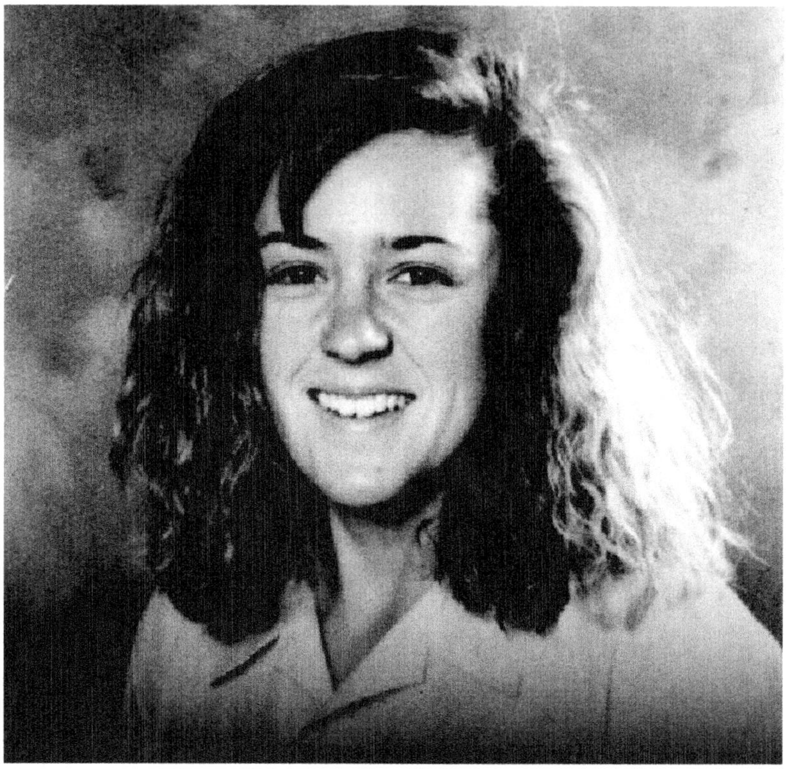

"The hospital psychiatrist gave me a great bit of advice. "Cancer is a high-maintenance illness." He said, "People will be coming at least every four hours to check you, so they know what's happening in your body." I felt, "Okay, cool. I've got it." That was a massive help to know that all this relentless activity was normal."

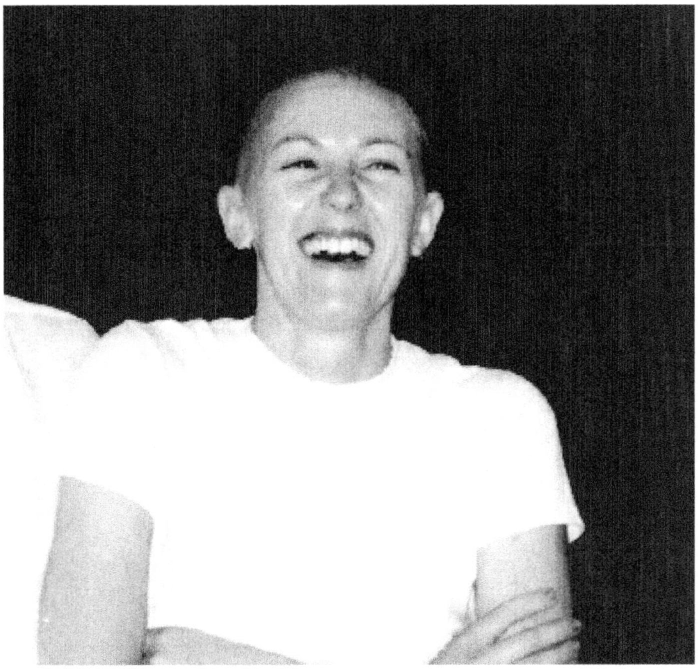

"One thing cancer gave me was a superb bullshit detector. I remember having a conversation with my uncle who had had a couple of heart attacks, and he said, "Being faced with your own mortality makes you realise what's important in life and what's bullshit."

One day when she was 27, Mel Cain showed her mum some bruises she'd noticed on her legs. Her mother, who had been the secretary for a paediatrician for 12 years and had seen those bruises many times before, sent her straight off to the doctors. Mel was diagnosed with acute promyelocytic leukemia – an aggressive and fast acting cancer – on the Thursday and was told 'Get your things together, you're in hospital from Monday.' She underwent eight months of treatment and at one stage got so ill that she saw the look on her mum's face that said, 'I think my daughter is going to die'. Now in remission, Mel is 40, married and living in Los Angeles with her husband, RP, and their naturally conceived daughter, Lola.

"Everybody in the hospital is there to help you. So listen and ask questions, even if you're scared of the answers – you have to do it."

DR CHARLIE TEO

"Brain cancer is the most aggressive of all cancers. It's the number one killer of males between the ages of 35 and 45, and the number one killer of children. If people realised how little money is put into neurosurgery, and especially brain cancer research, I think they'd be quite shocked and pretty upset."

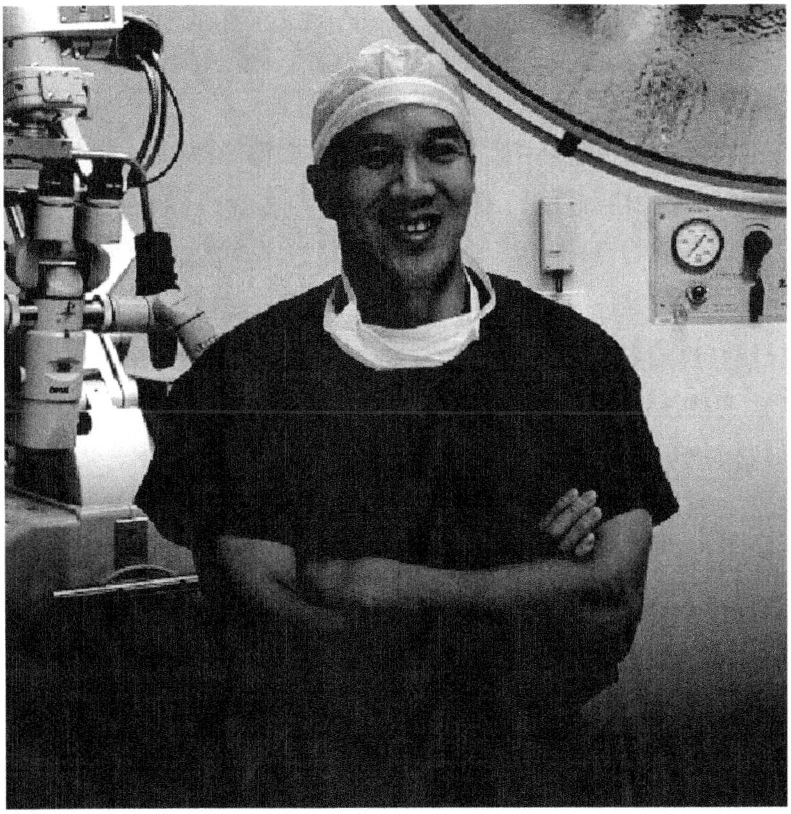

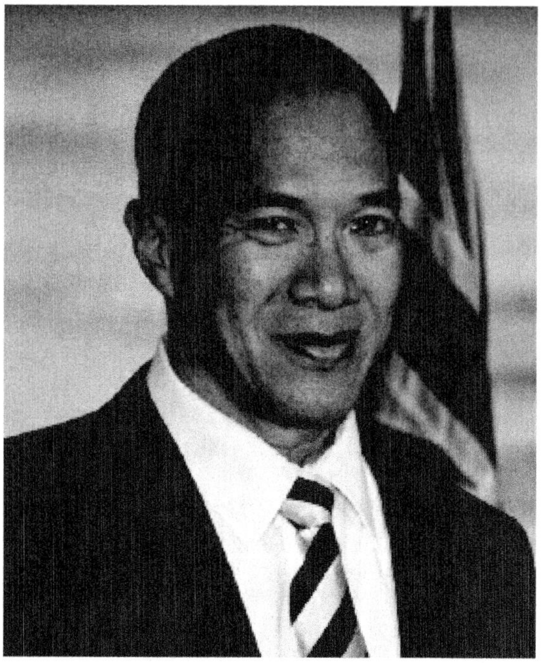

"Ask yourself, "Are you prepared to die or do you really want to cling on to life?" We all get three quotes to fix our cars. Why don't we get three quotes when diagnosed with cancer? Unfortunately people blindly accept the first diagnosis they receive. To beat a formidable foe, you have to be equally as aggressive and powerful. So you need to find a doctor who is going to be proactive, who's going to be aggressive and who's going to treat this cancer the way it ought to be treated."

Dr Charlie Teo, 53, is the Director of the Centre for Minimally Invasive Neurosurgery; Founder of the Cure for Life Foundation; Associate Professor of Neurosurgery at the University of New South Wales. He specialises in the treatment of adult and childhood brain tumours. The techniques and skills he offers have saved or extended the lives of many children from both Australia and abroad, who have been diagnosed with so-called 'inoperable' brain tumours.

"Avoid near field radiation, given off by electricity. As a rough guide, don't let anything electrical within one arm's length of your brain. Keep computers one arm's length away, don't leave the electric blanket on when you're in bed and turn off any electrical cords near your head at night. You'd be foolish to sleep in a position where there is a fuse box on the other side of the wall."

TONY CARR

"Be very, very diligent when you're listening to your specialist. If you have any worries or doubts, get a second opinion."

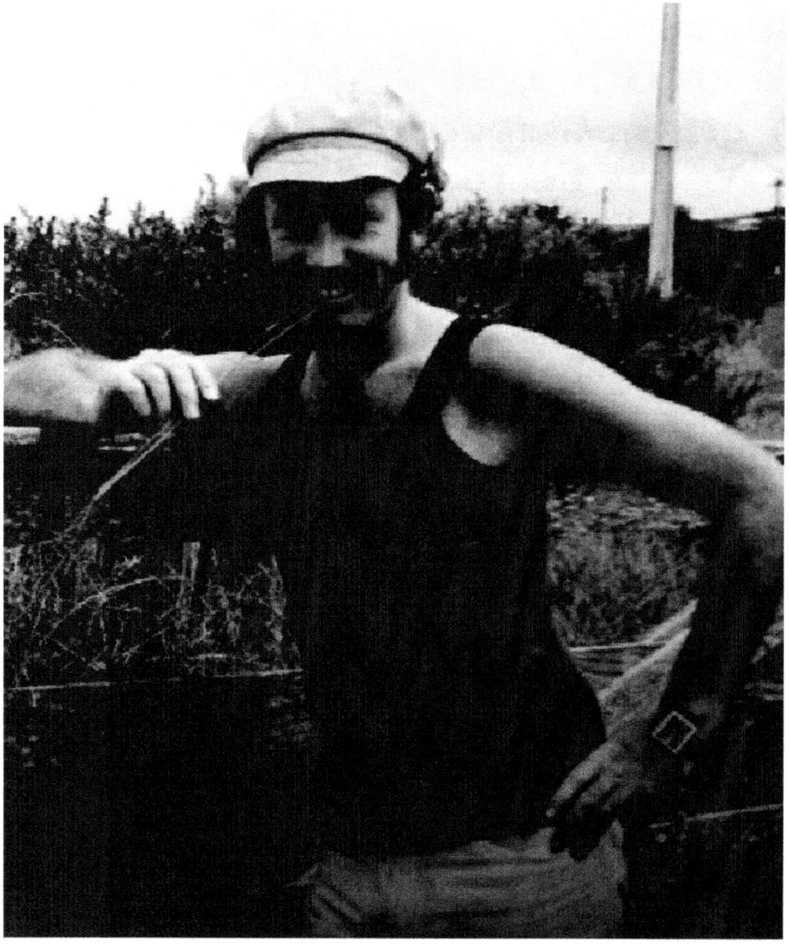

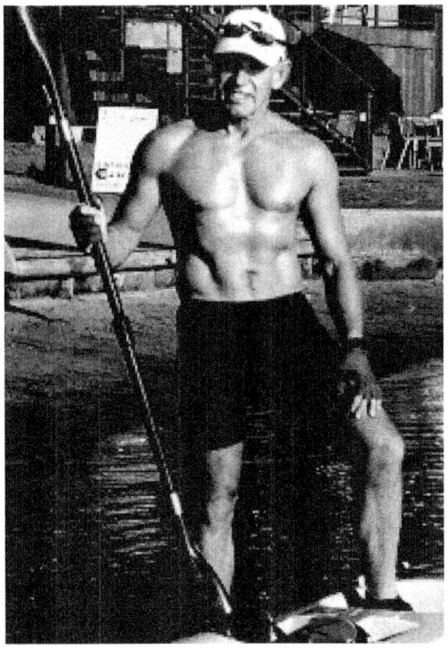

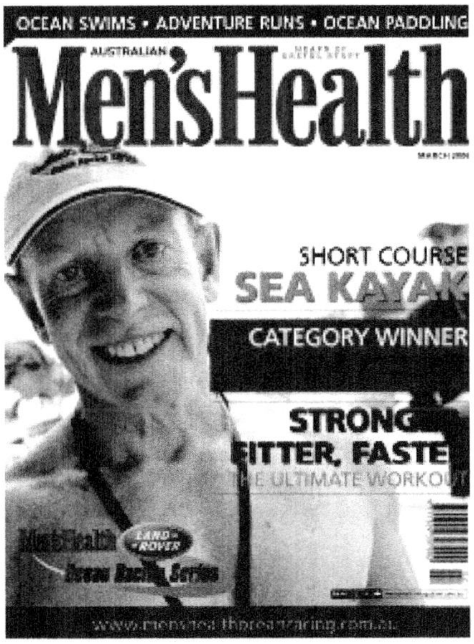

When his PSA levels – an indicator for prostate cancer-kept going up, Tony Carr, 68, saw a specialist who did biopsies then looked him in the eye and said, 'You do not have cancer'. After six months of his PSA rising further, he saw another specialist who did more biopsies – this time from both sides of the prostate

– and the diagnosis was different. Tony had surgery for prostate cancer.

"Pay much more attention to unusual symptoms. I lived with an ache in my back for far too long. After a month I should have gone to the GP and said, "This is not right." But I waited six or eight months and kept thinking "Oh, this will go away." And that was stupid."

One day, a few years after his prostate cancer, Tony lent forward in a Yoga class and felt an excruciating pain in his back. He had non-Hodgkin's lymphoma eating through his ribs, and the pain was one of his weakened bone snapping.

"You should maintain a healthy lifestyle anyway, but especially if you're going to have surgery or chemo. Take the time to get really fit even if it means you have to delay the chemo or the surgery a bit because you'll get through it much better and bounce back really quickly."

Enthusiastic kayaker, Tony won the *Men's Health Magazine* Ocean Racing series-and a Landrover Discovery – while he was in the middle of his course of chemotherapy for non-Hodgkin's lymphoma. He laughs and says 'Well, they didn't ask if I'd taken any "performance decreasing drugs"'.

CHRISSIE KEEPENCE

"Over the last several years researchers have discovered that mutations in the genes, BRCA 1 or BRCA 2, give you up to an 80 percent chance of developing breast cancer. The odds are pretty high. If I had those odds on winning blackjack, I'd be in the casino every night. When my sisters and I found out we had the mutated gene, we knew we had to act on it."

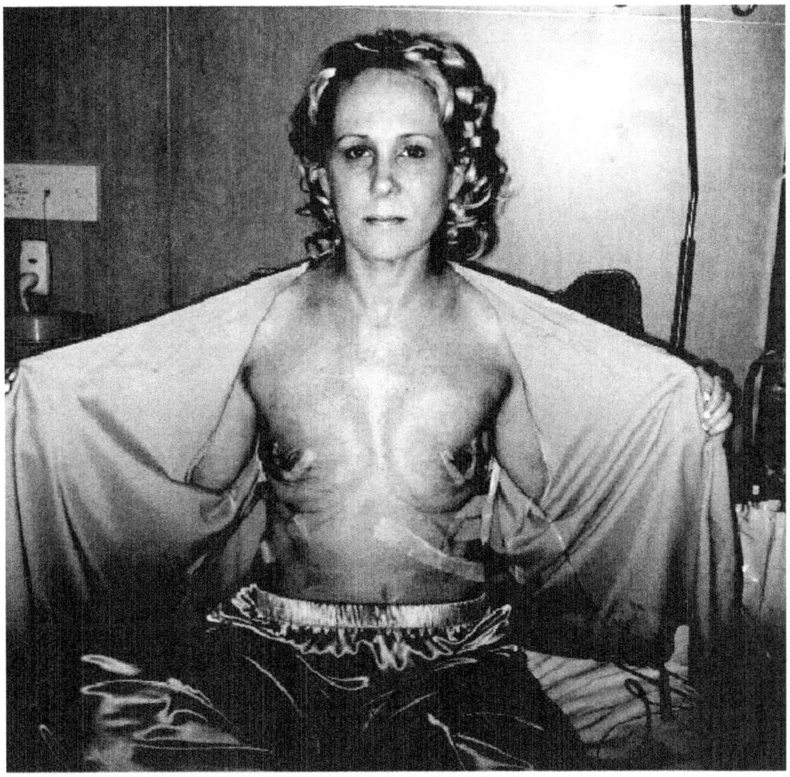

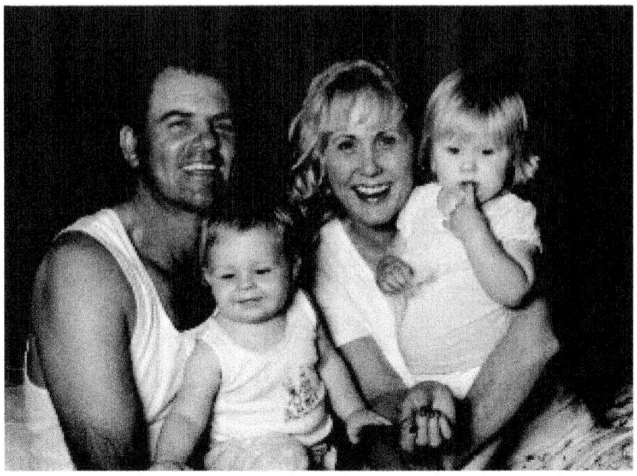

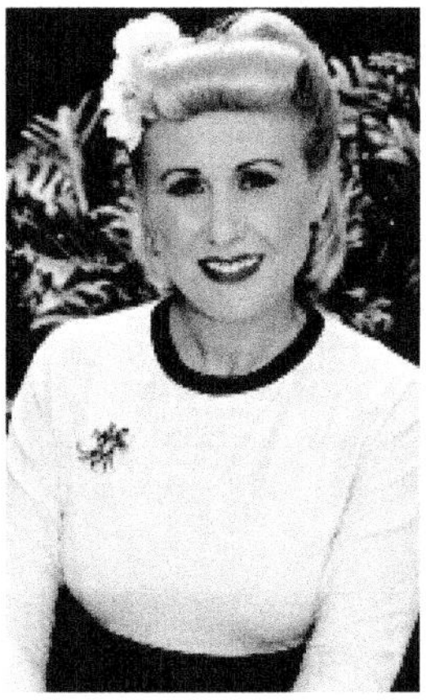

"The physical pain and limitations associated with having a prophylactic mastectomy for me lasted about six months. Compared to a lifetime of prevention, anxiety, worry, and knowing that one day you may get cancer, or decide to remove your breasts to prevent it anyway, I decided to have the operation and eliminate the uncertainty. For me it was short-term pain for long term gain."

I tell myself that I'm lucky and I say to women identified with BRCA 1 or 2, "Don't look at this

as a death sentence. Try to see how lucky you are that you have this choice."

Chrissie Keepence, 45, is one of three sisters who had a history of breast cancer deaths in their family. When their mother was also diagnosed with breast cancer at 50 years old, the sisters decided they weren't prepared to take any chances with their own lives. They found a genetic research program that identifies whether you have the gene marker for breast cancer, and they were all tested – and all were positive. Chrissie decided, virtually on the spot, to have both her breasts removed, and she is now also about to undergo a hysterectomy.

When you're a woman with cancer, there's an abundance of information and support, and so there should be. But when you're in the position my sisters and I found ourselves in – as a pre-vivor, or someone who is almost certainly going to get cancer – the support isn't quite there yet. No-one knows about it.

WENDY STARKIE

"Don't run around saying "Oh God, Oh God. Why me? What have I done wrong?" There are no answers to those questions, so don't waste your energy – you don't have any to spare. The only thing you can control is how you react to the situation."

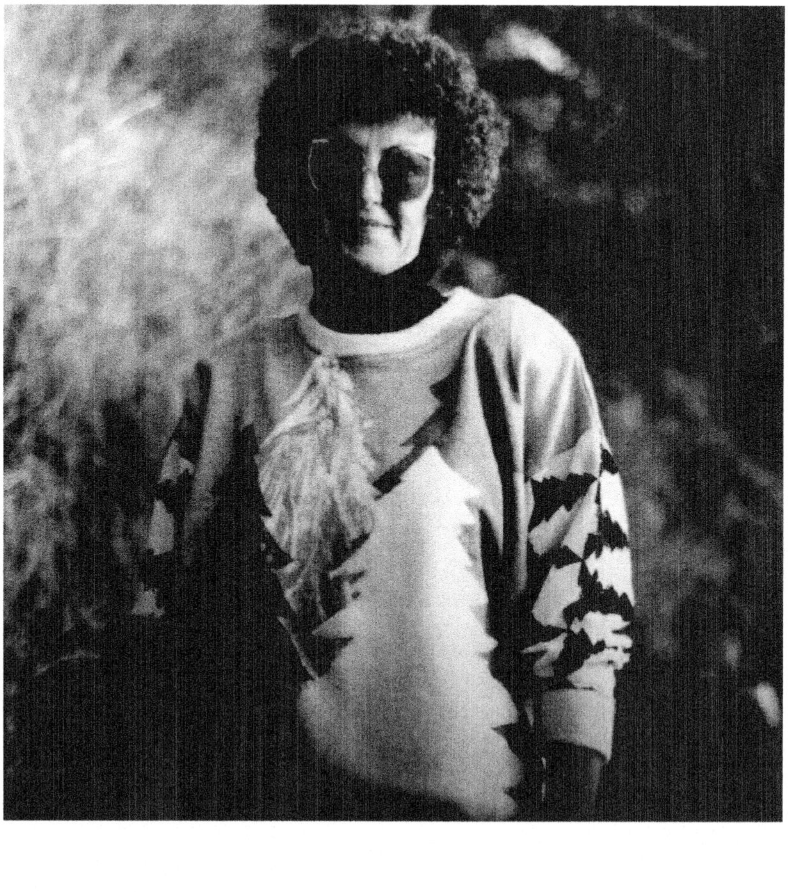

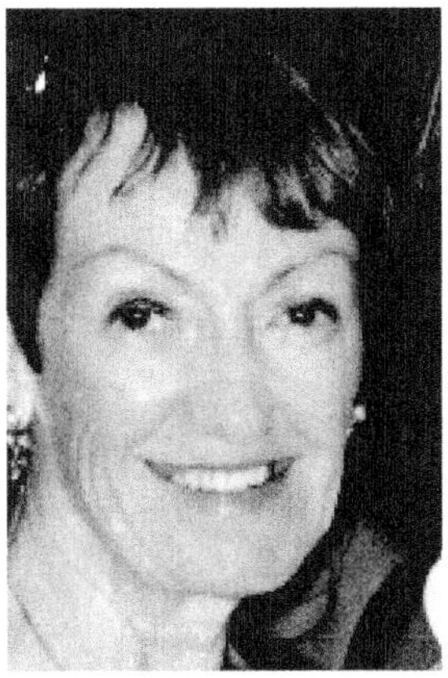

"Cancer taught me how wonderful life is, and how wonderful the world is. You realise how fleeting our time is here, how easily life is snuffed out, and how much you must appreciate every single second of every day. Life is not a dress rehearsal. This is opening night every single day."

Wendy Starkie, 64, nursed her husband for 13 months as he died from a malignant brain tumour. Six months later she had a regular breast scan and was diagnosed with breast cancer. Wendy remembers being at a set of traffic lights and all this anger that had been building up exploded out of her as she hammered on the steering wheel and screamed out 'I will NOT die! YOU WON'T KILL ME!' She laughs as she recalls 'I looked around and everybody was staring at me open mouthed. The traffic lights had turned green but everyone was too scared to beep the horn to tell me to go.' Since her treatment Wendy has embraced life to the full. She has climbed Mt Kilimanjaro, started giving seminars on dealing with cancer, joined a gym and this year she won her local gym's 2010 Award for the most amazing results.

"Your friends really do want to help. When my husband had his cancer, he liked to keep life normal and we used to love entertaining, but I was too exhausted from looking after him to put together a dinner party. So I'd ring up friends and say, "Please come to dinner on Saturday night and bring the entree." Someone else would bring the main course, another couple would make the dessert, and I'd provide the wine. And we'd put a party together and my husband would sit there and say, "This is wonderful. It's just like there's nothing wrong, isn't it?"

"When you've had to look death in the face twice, as I have, you're not frightened of dying anymore. What you're frightened of is dying without achieving everything you wanted to do They said to me, "It will be dangerous up Mt Kilimanjaro." I said, "It's dangerous crossing the road in the middle of Sydney. And I'd rather die on top of Mt Kilimanjaro than in the middle of George Street."

SALLY MCAULIFFE

"Keep your family together during it. Don't underestimate how much the family unit is essential to the child that is going through treatment. Don't isolate them from the everyday."

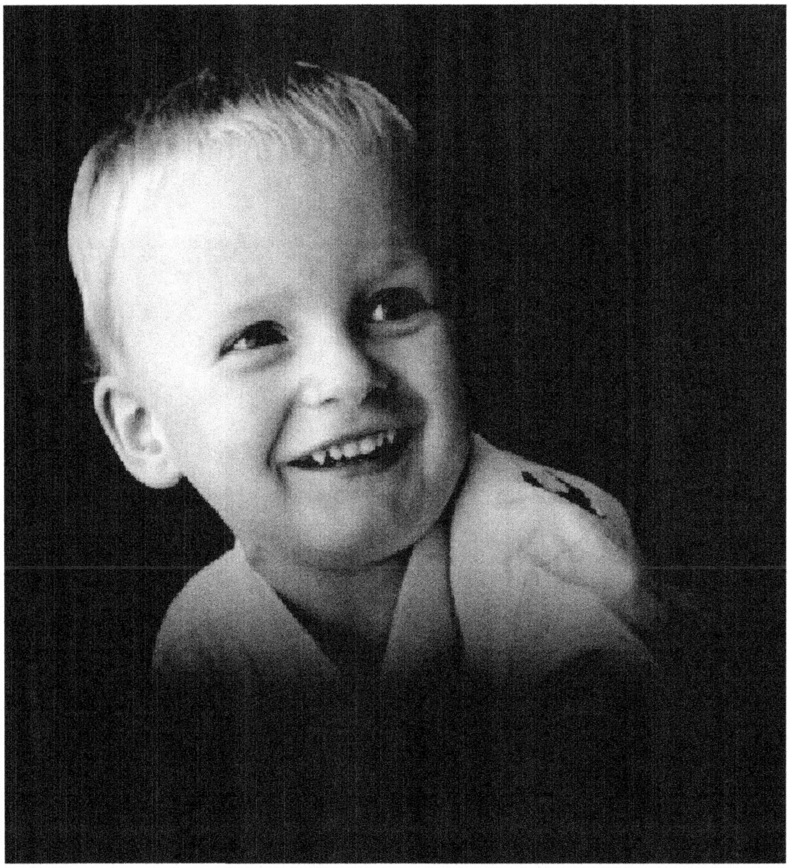

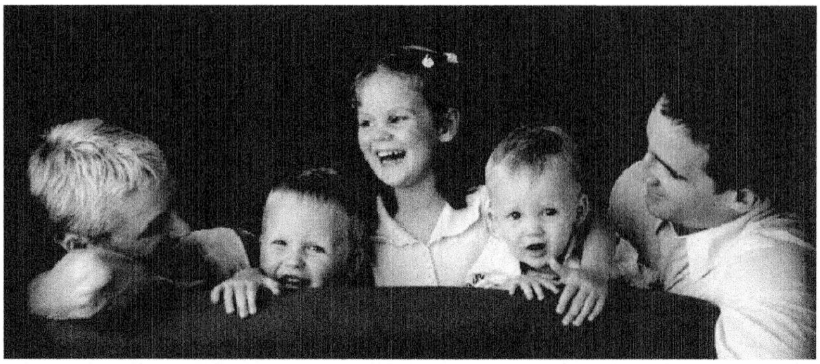

"I believe that you've got to keep the norm, which sounds bizarre, but cancer became our new norm. I'd go into Conor in the morning and he'd ask, "Are we going to the hospital today, mum?" and I'd say, "No mate, not today. Isn't that good?" And he'd reply, "But I like it there."

"You don't have to wrap them up in cotton wool and not let them have a life. I don't think Conor had a bad time during his 15 months of treatment. I think he was a very happy little boy. For him, cancer and its treatment were just normal life"

In 2005, life was as good as it could get for Sally and Mick McAuliffe. They were living in New Zealand, had two beautiful children and another on the way. They could never have predicted how their lives were about to change when their nearly two-year-old son, Conor, complained of a tummy ache one evening. It was found that Conor had stage four liver cancer and after 15 months of gruelling treatment, Sally and Mick's brave little boy lost his battle.

"They'd be riding bikes and he'd go and have a vomit from his chemo and then get back on his bike and keep going. I think kids go through cancer treatment very differently from an adult. Kids just get on with life. It's amazing to watch."

"Don't exclude yourselves from other parents going through it because they are the ones who get it. We spent a lot of time talking to other parents of kids with cancer at the time and that was a huge support."

Conor has taught us to let go of the little things. To hold on to what's important right now.

GEORGE KONIA

Cancer is not an automatic death sentence and, with a healthy attitude and good direction, little miracles can happen.

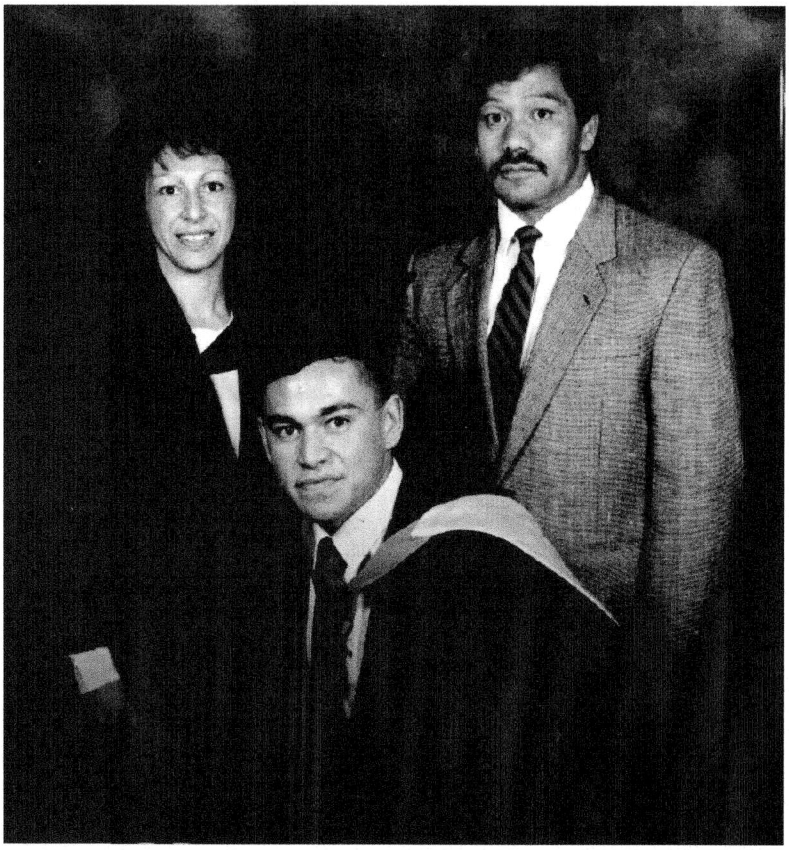

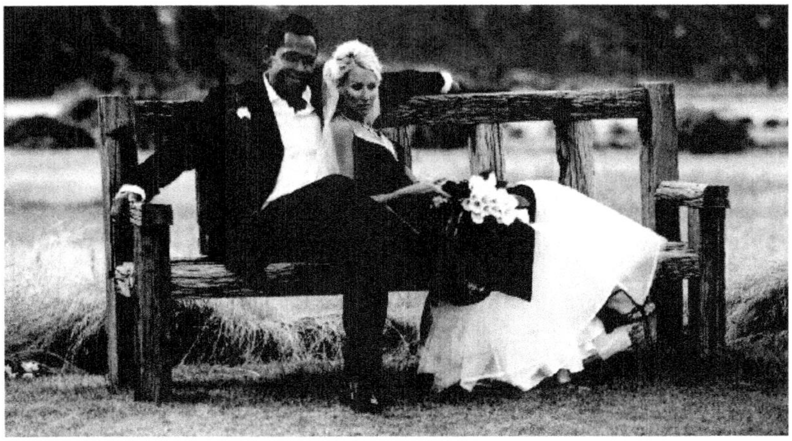

"Having cancer clarifies what is really important and what is not. It made me ask some searching questions of myself and my maker. It forced me to stop, slow down, and reassess where I really wanted to go and what I wanted to do."

George Konia, 41, was a group fitness instructor, a fitness centre manager, a personal trainer and was renovating properties after work. This meant he was starting work about 6 am, working through to about 2 or 3 am, then having a short nap and charging on again. Then he and his (then) girlfriend, Gena, were told George had Lymphoma. They went out to his car, gave each other a big hug and started to drive. The stereo blared out *The Scientist* by Coldplay, 'Nobody said it was easy ... Can we go back to the start?' and they cried all the way home. The song became their anthem, and George and Gena eventually used it as their wedding song three years later. The couple now have a gorgeous two-year-old daughter, Scarlett, who was fathered naturally, much to his doctors' surprise and their delight. To celebrate five years since his bone marrow transplant, George recently did the Wanaka Iron Man in New Zealand.

Be mindful of how much your partner is hurting. As a cancer patient you have no choice but to deal with whatever the doctors throw at you, but your partner has no idea what you are going through, how they can help, or whether you are even going to make it. They can feel totally helpless. It must be incredibly hard to watch the one you love deteriorate right in front of your eyes and not be able to do a bloody thing about it.

CHRIS BLAMEY

"When it comes to stress at work, you have to start making your own rules. Set your own agenda. Our MD was quite good; he would turn his phone off at 8 o'clock on Friday nights. That was it. These days phone calls come through at any hour of the day or night, and you're just expected to be available."

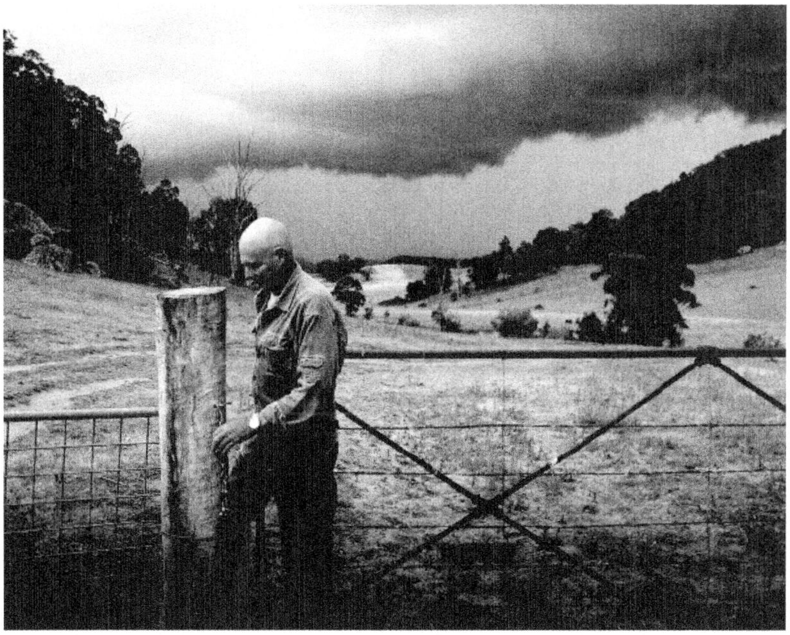

Chris Blamey, 64, smoked until the eighties, worked an incredibly busy week at a stressful job where he often travelled and then flew home on the weekend to run the 2000 acre family farm. While the farm work was very busy, Chris found it relaxing – it was out of mobile reception – he is now convinced he didn't take enough care handling farm chemicals. Chris was diagnosed with non-Hodgkin's lymphoma when they found a lump in his chest the size of a football, and underwent chemo and radiotherapy. Now he is in remission, keeps his weight down, tries to avoid taking too much on and almost never uses chemicals on his farm, or anywhere else – he's even stopped dying his hair.

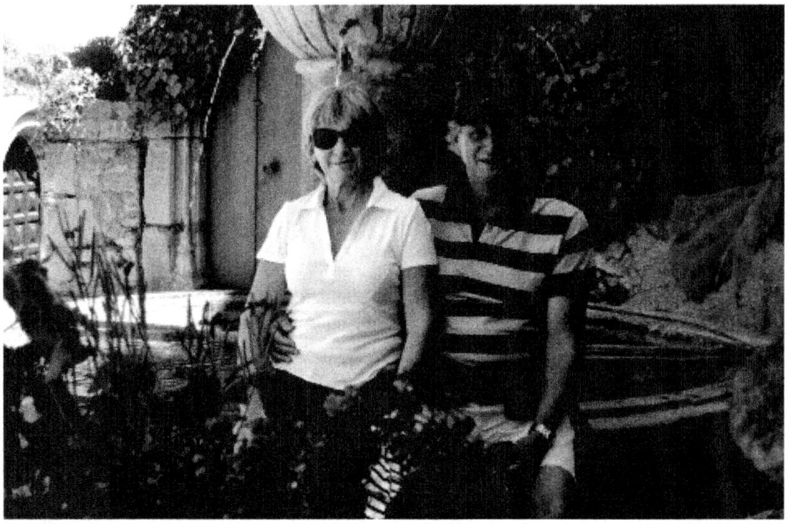

"I worked in a rural farming company and everyone there kept stressing that, when handling chemicals, masks, long rubber gloves and plastic pants need to be worn, to make sure that nothing penetrates the skin. I wish now that I'd persevered in getting Chris to handle the farm chemicals more safely, particularly when I saw his skin getting blotchy and red."

Ann Blamey, 63, would advise people to be prepared to feel incredibly frustrated looking after someone during their cancer treatment as it's hard to know how to help. She says you have to realise in the end there are times when, no matter how much you care, you can't really do anything.

"Since Dad's cancer I've made changes to my life. I keep as healthy as I can, and even when I'm away with work I still get up and go for a run or a walk on the beach. Now I also take an hour a day just to sit by myself and reflect on the big picture. And, during that time, things that I thought were huge issues invariably don't seem so big anymore."

Looking back, Chris's son, Jarrod, could see it was all too much for his Dad, but at the time he thought Chris was just 'doing what dads do' and didn't realise how much all this stress was affecting him. Now, even though Jarrod runs a huge company himself, he always tries to turn off his mobile on Friday afternoons.

CALLAN BACK

"No amount of watching House, seeing Cancer Council ads, or hearing stories from friends can ever prepare you for the emotions that tear through every inch of you as you suddenly realise: "Holy shit. I have cancer."

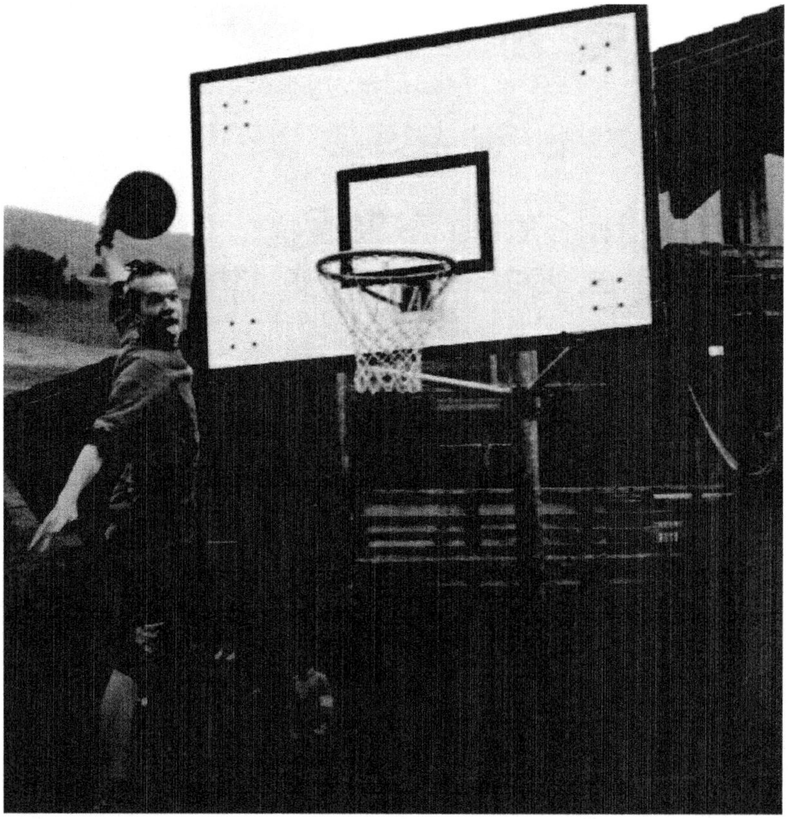

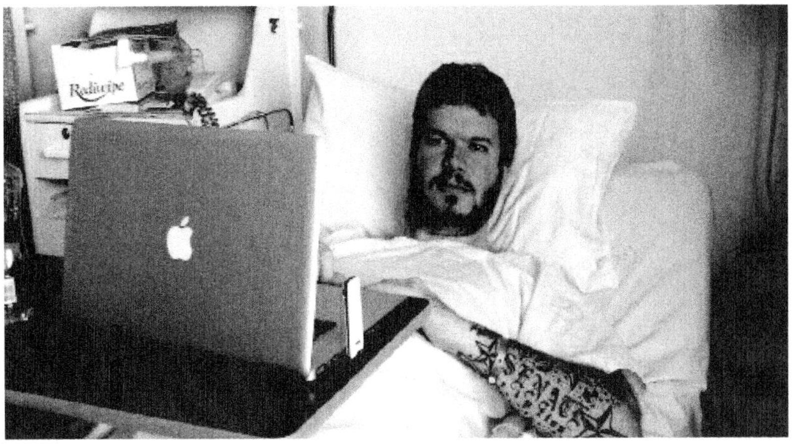

"Humour has gotten me through this ordeal. My favourite is to use really inappropriate excuses in everyday situations. If someone needs me to help out with the dishes I say, "I'd really love to, but you know, the cancer..." Some people think it's wrong, to make a joke out of it, but I just say "I'm sorry. It's not me, it's the cancer..."

Callan Back, age 31, has always been (and still is) your stereotypical computer geek. In his own words he 'sees so little sun that I'm practically translucent' – so he figured skin cancer was the last things he had to worry about. Then, one day, his wife, Irene, who is a nurse, noticed that a mole on his left thigh had puffed up. They went to the local doctor, then a dermatologist who diagnosed it as melanoma, and booked Callan in straight away to have it cut out. The cancer had spread to his lymph nodes and now, five surgeries later, they think they got the last of it. Callan is now in the middle of treatment with Interferon.

"Get regular checkups at a local clinic. It only takes half an hour. Finding something early is the difference between a one hour clinic visit and four months in and out of hospital getting surgeries, losing pieces of your body, and being crippled for the rest of your life."

"The biggest surprise has been how little I knew about nodular melanoma. How many of us know how easily a little mole can become a melanoma that spreads through the lymphatic system and end up in your brain, lungs, or other parts of your body? How many of us know that you can get melanoma from too LITTLE sun?"

"Cancer is not just something that smokers, tanners, and old people get. Understand that a balanced, healthy life could probably have prevented all this hell that I am going through now."

NERYS CHEESEBROUGH

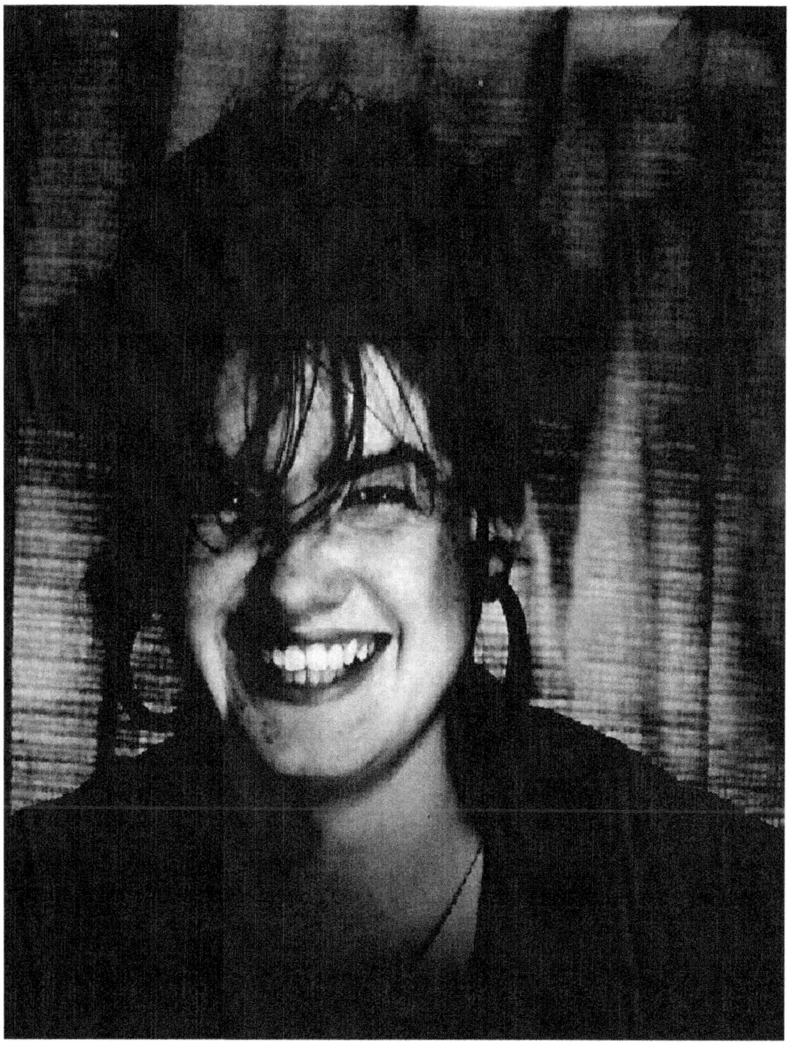

Chemotherapy has been vicious and evil, but absolutely necessary. It's everything you read about: poisonous, toxic, sickening and nasty. You willingly have the fluid pumped into your veins which makes every part of you scream in pain. The loss of hair, eyebrows and eyelashes (and

some of my nails) was the toughest part. All your identity is stripped, and you're left with a bloated person you no longer recognise. So, when you're going into it, understand that chemo hurts physically and scars mentally.

"Be prepared to laugh at the funny things that happen. One time I caught myself outside in a stripey top and my bandana. And I realised that all I needed was an eye-patch and a parrot. *Ah-harrrr, Jim Lad!*"

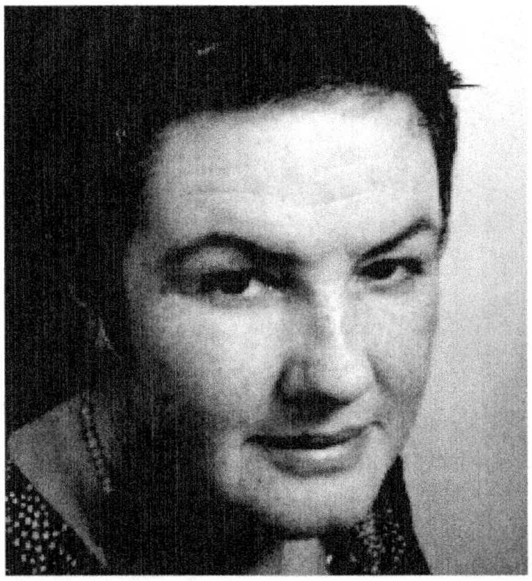

"Cancer and its treatment is a LONG, LONG, LONG process. It's not just diagnosis+treatment=cure. I was once told it was like peeling an onion. Every time I went back to the specialist we'd peel another layer, and more often than not I'd cry!"

Nerys Cheesebrough, 45, says that her experience with breast cancer taught her that some people really can't deal with such a big illness and have difficulty talking about 'it'. However she also believes that it's absolutely fine to rant/swear/whinge when you want to, as you can't 'be brave' all the time. Your close friends and family WILL understand when you scream and cry until your eyes are sore, your body hurts and you're 'too exhausted to be nice'.

NICOLE STEERS

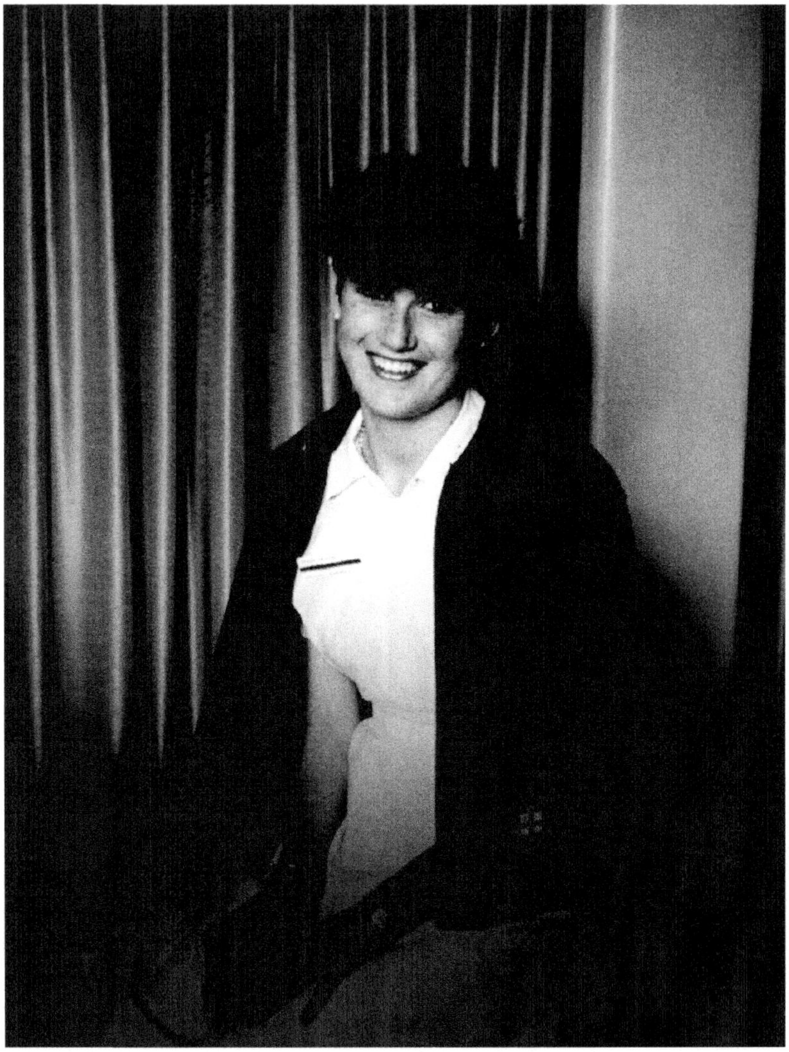

"I would say to all health professionals that we need to listen more to our clients and their families. Just because you can do task one to ten for them doesn't mean you should. The patient might only want one small thing from you, or they might want a whole multitude. They

might need you to talk to their GP or other health professional, or they might want to include their families. One man I looked after just needed help navigating the health system. We all have to remember to ask the patient how they want things to go. After all it really is their call."

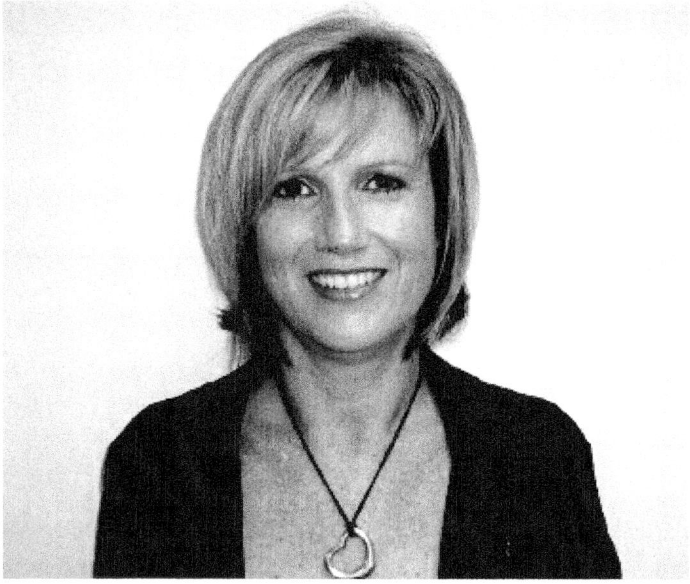

"When I worked as a Breast Care Nurse, spouses would often say to me, "I just feel so helpless", I just want to take their pain away, or even share the pain, but I can't. Often partners really need something tangible to do, so if a patient needs an injection three times a day, I'd ask the partner if they would like to learn how to do that. Then they know they're making a difference. On the other hand, some people prefer to let professional carers do the caring,

so the partner can remain a partner, a lover, a friend or whatever, which is sometimes all the patient wants."

As a registered nurse Nicole Steers had opportunity to work as Nurse Counsellor for BreastScreen which opened up many doors. She ended up as a Breast Care Nurse and eventually moved into management having responsibility for cancer services in a regional centre, which led to other opportunities in the inpatient and community settings whilst maintaining a cancer and palliative care focus.

PAULA MCCAFFREY

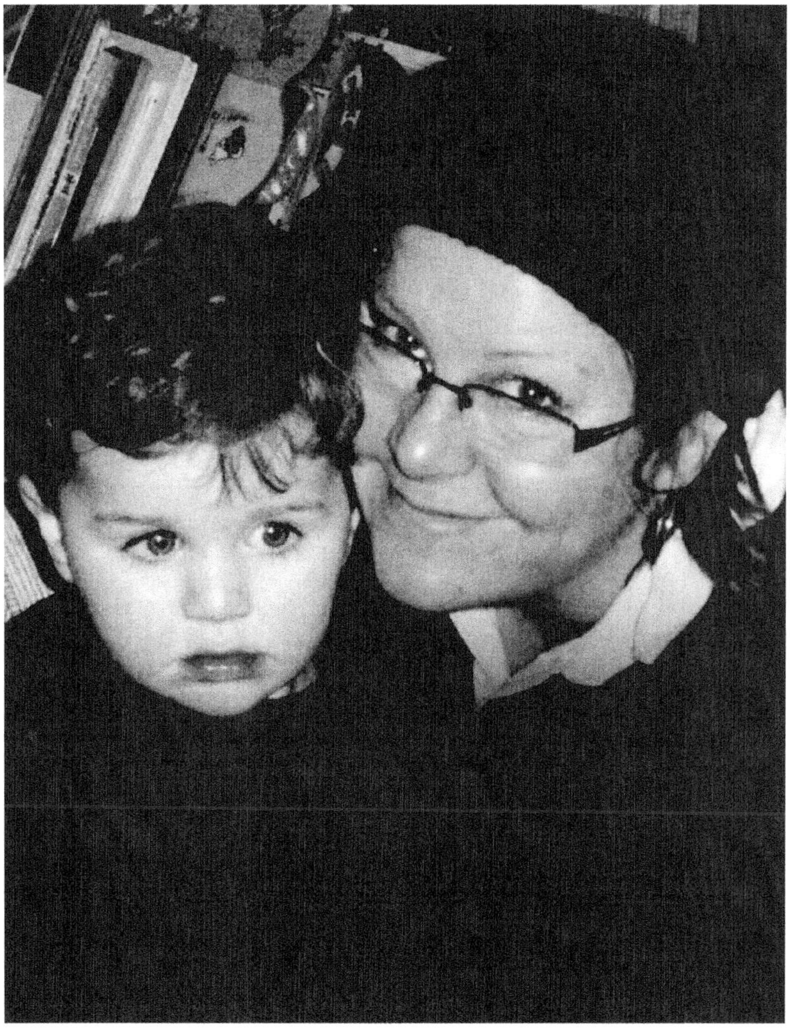

"I relied on the mantra, "This too shall pass", and found it incredibly helpful because there were days when I felt so bad I was surviving second by second. The nausea, the headache and the fear. Then I thought, "This too shall pass." Those last few seconds have gone, I can make

it through the next few seconds, and then the next, and the next. Then you realise you've made it to the end of another day."

"Find reasons to live. For me it was my children. I want to see them go to school, I want to see their next birthdays ... I can't picture my life without them and I don't want to imagine their life without me."

After having some irregular bowel problems, Paula McCaffrey, 38, thought that she might have a gluten intolerance. When she finally had an x-ray and then a colonoscopy, she had tumour the size of a grapefruit obstructing her bowels. The cancer had gone through her bowel wall and into lymph and blood vessels, and Paula remembers being terrified and thinking 'God, I'm only 35 and I might not be here this time next year.' Paula had surgery which was excruciatingly painful, and resulted in an ileostomy – which meant she had to wear a bag to collect her waste for a few months – and eight cycles of chemotherapy. She says that her kids knew she wasn't well, and that even though her youngest child was only eighteen months old at that time, he wasn't smiling in any photos during her period of surgery and treatment.

"Handle it head on. I made a deliberate point of looking at myself in the mirror, at the 47cm wound in my abdomen, and at my ileostomy, then saying to myself, "I look beaten up, but I

can make this work. I am strong enough to do this."

"I'm supremely grateful for normal and won't ever, ever take it for granted again. Just being healthy, and having a husband, a house, a job, two beautiful children, wonderful parents and friends is an incredible gift. When you realise how easily you can lose it all, these things become incredibly special and you finally get that you don't really need any more than that. This doesn't mean you can't strive for more, but you don't *need* more."

MEREDITH HOPE

"A bit of black humour can go a long way. I remember talking to my husband about the lump on my toe. Without batting an eyelid he said, "Hmm, probably a metastasis." Strangely enough, this made me laugh and really helped."

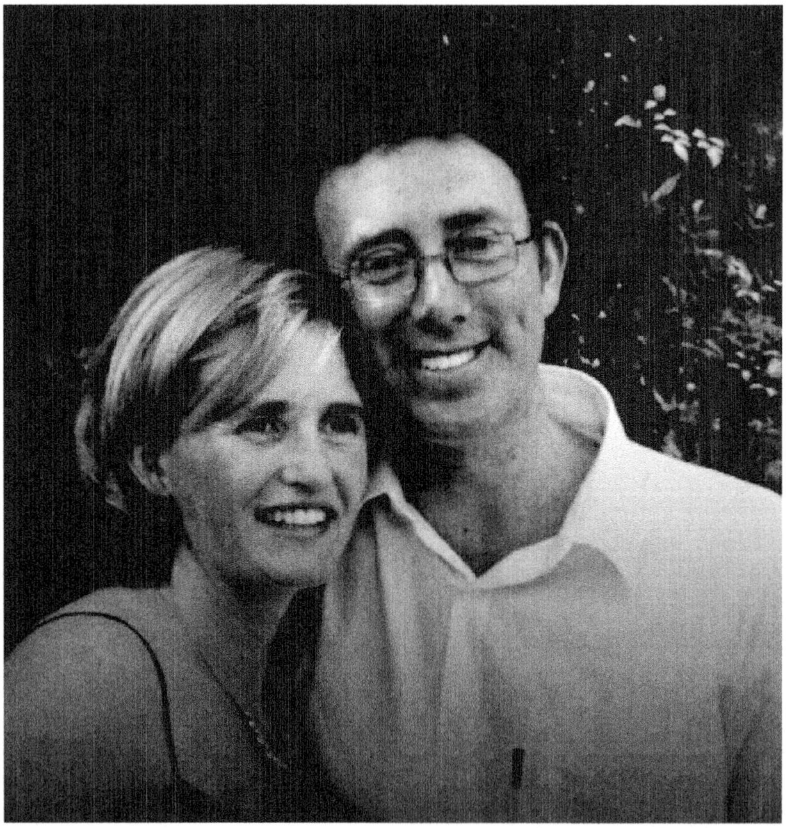

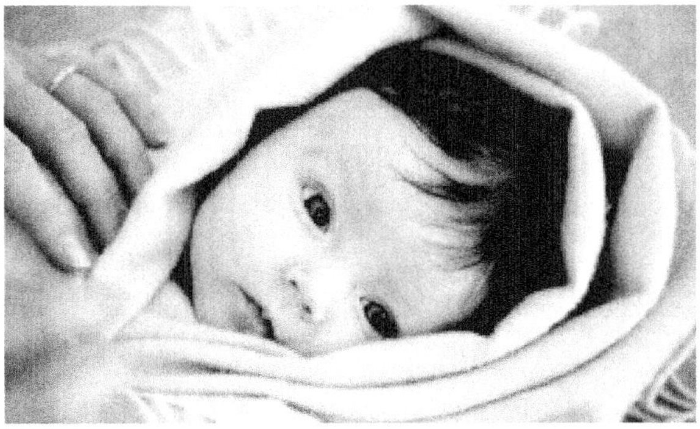

"Beware of people who want to judge you, or say things like "You brought this on yourself." I think these people are just wanting to separate themselves from those who are sick, so they don't have to face illness and their own mortality. One person actually said to me that I'd picked my genes, manifested this somehow, and chosen to have breast cancer. When you are vulnerable and in pain, others' judgement is the last thing you need. I just wanted my friends and family to hold my hand and walk through the darkness with me. On reflection, this capacity is rare but one of the most important gifts you can give to someone who is ill."

"Surround yourself with good counsel. Contain your fears by talking about them. If you spend all your time worrying about this pain or that lump, and not letting anyone know, you lose time and valuable energy. I had a wonderful GP who was a great help. At one stage I said, "I think I have toe cancer." My doctor said, "No, that's a corn."

Six weeks before her wedding, Meredith Hope, 39, discovered a lump in her breast while playing with her daughter, Sophie. She had her first course of chemotherapy just two weeks before the big day and spent her wedding night at hospital with an infection in her arm. Since then she has been given the 'five year, all clear' and – with her husband James – has celebrated the birth of their second daughter, Lucinda.

"The positive thinking movement has hairs on it. Blindly being positive because you're constantly told that this will get you well makes it impossible to talk about the hard realities. You need to hold the good and bad together. Work through the hard stuff – like wills and making videos for the child you might be about to leave behind – because if you don't, it plays on your mind, eats away at you and stops you being able to be truly positive."

"Try to find peace. Let go of the things you can't change. Find ways to say, "Thank you" to special people and "sorry" when it's needed. Bottled up bad feelings eat away at you and rob you of valuable energy. Peace is everything. It may not make you physically better but it can make every moment better. And finally, do things that give you joy and that you are passionate about. Joy and passion feed the soul and make each moment rich and fulfilling."

RENE MICHELL

"Do whatever makes you happy. Have as much happiness in your days as you can. Live your dreams, don't wait. Today is today, and that's all we have. Everyone only has right now. No one knows how long they have left."

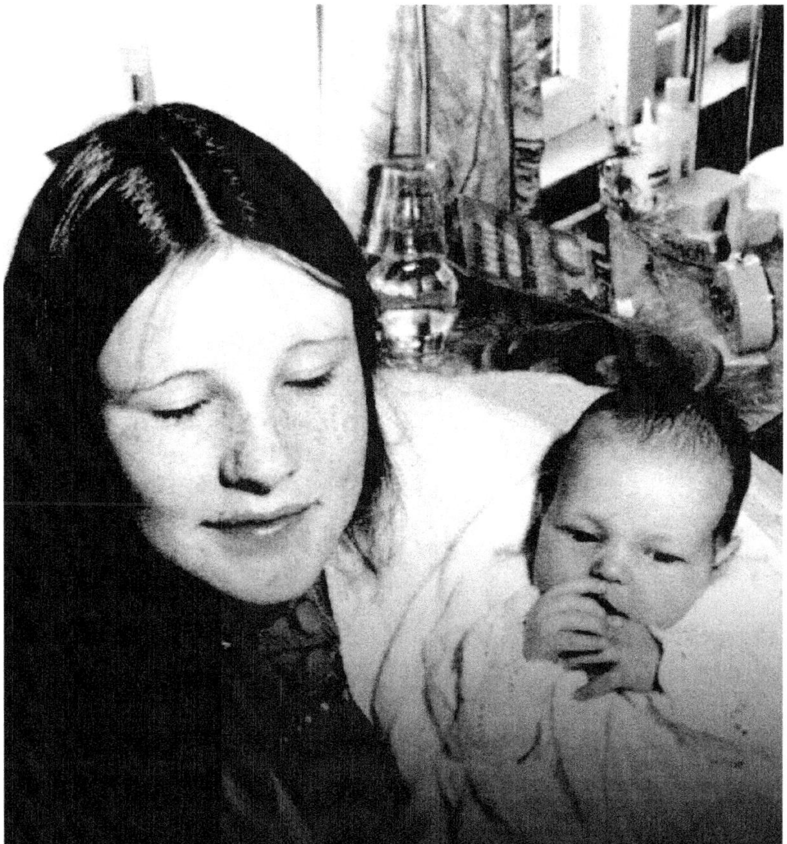

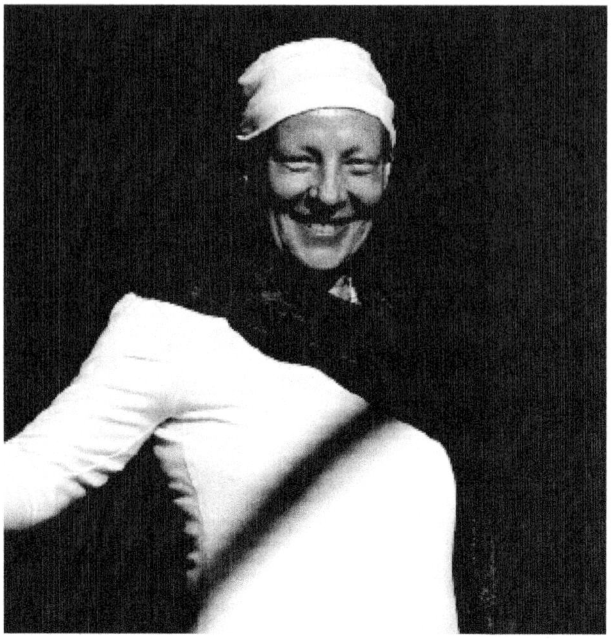

"Do as much healing as you can on yourself. Look deep within and see if you have held resentments and not forgiven people. I had been holding resentments towards my husband, and was holding back in many relationships. So now, even though I'm in the middle of treatment for cancer, I'm the happiest I've ever been."

–Sometimes people will say the wrong thing, and you have to just let it go.

Rene Michell, 54, remembers leaving hospital for the first time when she was just starting treatment for ovarian cancer, and a doctor saying to her 'You know, you'll probably die from this.' Rene quickly replied 'Well, you'll probably get hit by a bus, but what are you gonna do?' At the time she didn't like it at all, but later Rene later thanked the woman – in her mind at least – because it gave her so much drive to fight it and prove her wrong.

"Find a positive person you can talk to about anything, then download. I was pretty scared and just wanted someone to send me a lifeline and get me out of here, though I knew that wasn't possible. So find a person who is not promising anything, someone who can just listen."

MARGARET GRAY

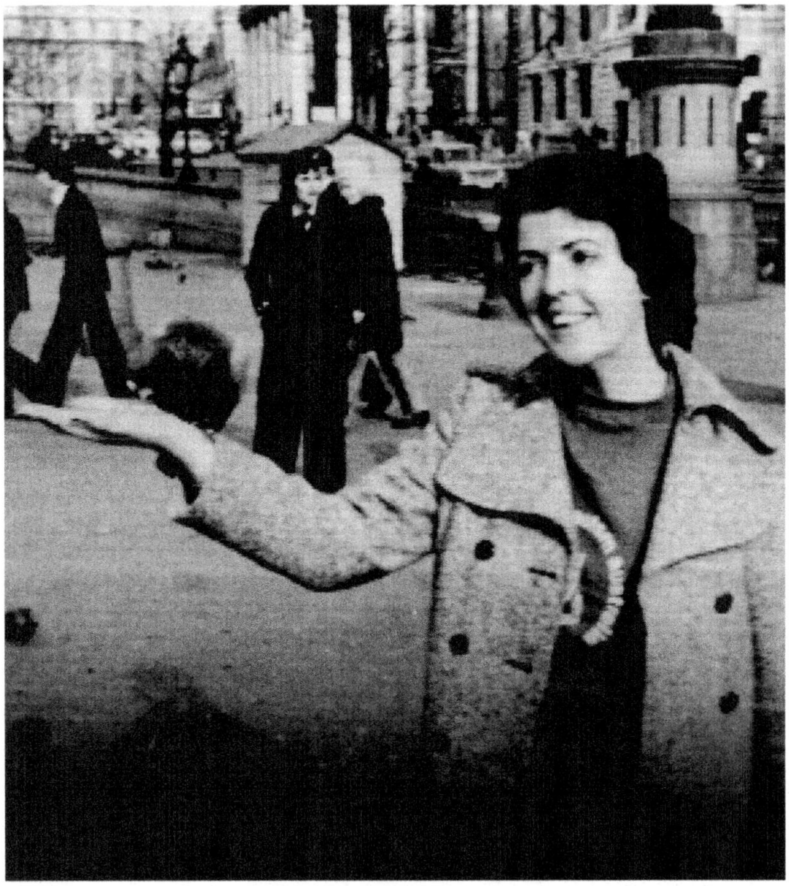

"The decision about what to do should be down to the person who has the cancer. Listen to everyone, but remember that oncologists, surgeons, radiologists, even friends and family – while all incredibly well intentioned – have their own agenda."

If you don't totally trust your doctor, change them. It's nothing personal, you just have to get

someone you feel absolutely comfortable putting your life in their hands, because that's exactly what you're doing.

Margaret Gray, 58, says that when she was diagnosed with breast cancer she listened to the advice, opinions and concerns of others, got information about the various options, their costs and disruption to her life, and eventually she was very comfortable with her decision to have a mastectomy, but not the suggested chemotherapy. Margaret says 'They told me there was a 30% chance it would come back in 10 years, but I saw that as a 70% chance that it wouldn't!'.

Take it all one step at a time. Get as much information as you need before you give anybody the go ahead for any treatment. It's rarely so urgent that you can't take some time to have a few deep breaths and think about your options.

BRUCE SULLIVAN

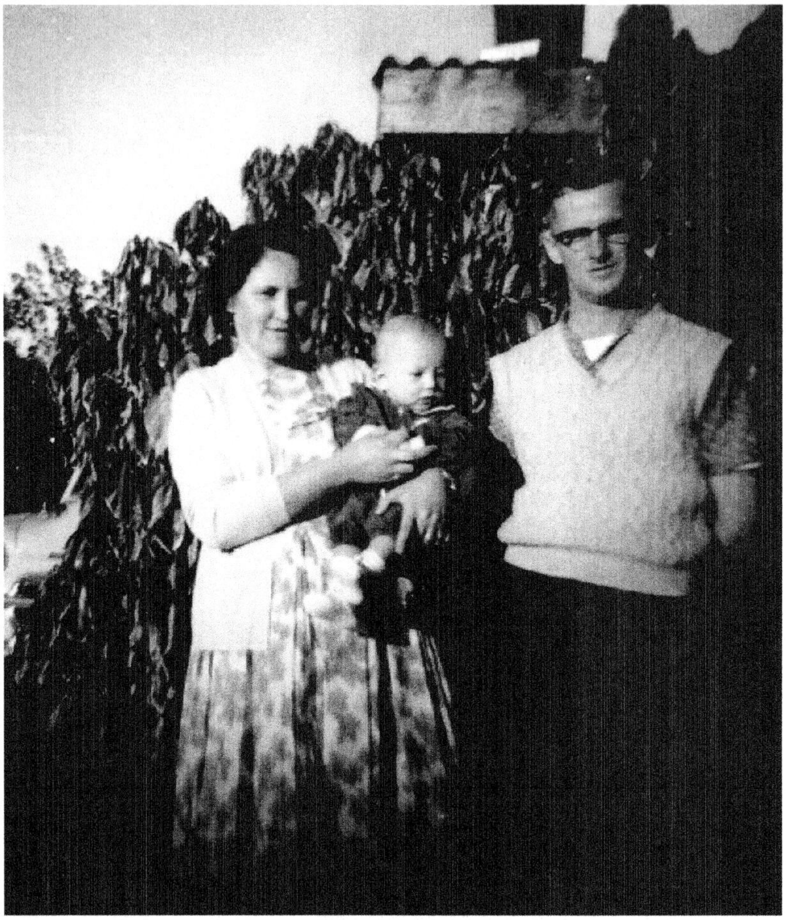

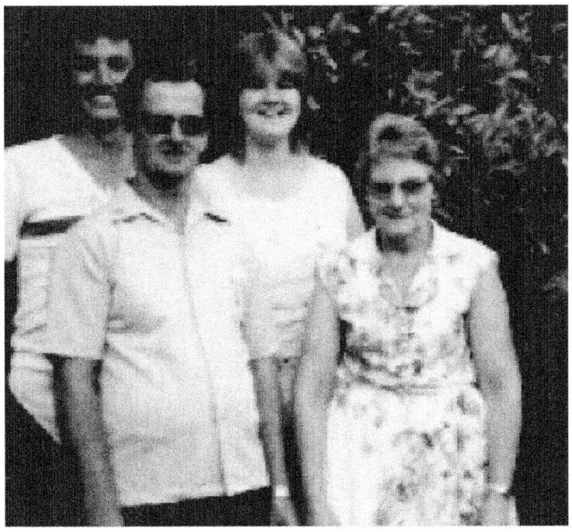

"When someone in your family is dealing with cancer, you'll start to feel like you just can't pick up that telephone and go through the whole update one more time. So leave a good long message on your answering machine like "G'day. It's Monday, three o'clock. Thanks for calling but we're either looking after Mum or resting ourselves. Here's the latest..." that type of thing. Then update it often because people crave information."

When someone you know has cancer, don't ask if they need your help, just go and lend a hand They'll probably say, "No it's all good." So just go and help – fold their laundry, mow their lawn, just pitch in. Then go around to the people looking after the person with cancer and cut their grass too. Care for the carers.

When he was in his late teens Bruce Sullivan, now 45, remembers his mum being treated for breast cancer. After he finished Year 12 – partly because his mother seemed okay, and partly because she insisted he go – he went off on a holiday. On the third day he called home from the local phone box and the phone rang unanswered – something totally unheard of in his house. When he eventually got hold of someone he learned that his mum had lapsed into a coma and died. To this day he believes that, if someone had been telling him exactly what was really going on, he would have stayed at home.

"The thing I learned is that when someone else dies there is the physical transition, where you watch this person go from being a healthy person to their eminent death. Just as important for you is the emotional transition. A lot of people just hope this will take care of itself. Some cultures do grief incredibly well, with good structure that gives people permission to mourn, then even if you don't feel like it you wail for your husband one more day because you've got to do the wailing for three days. In Australia we don't give people enough permission to grieve."

ANDREW MAY

"You know when you're busy and you think you've got a lot on? When you hear the words "You've got cancer", suddenly you're not so busy. It puts everything into perspective."

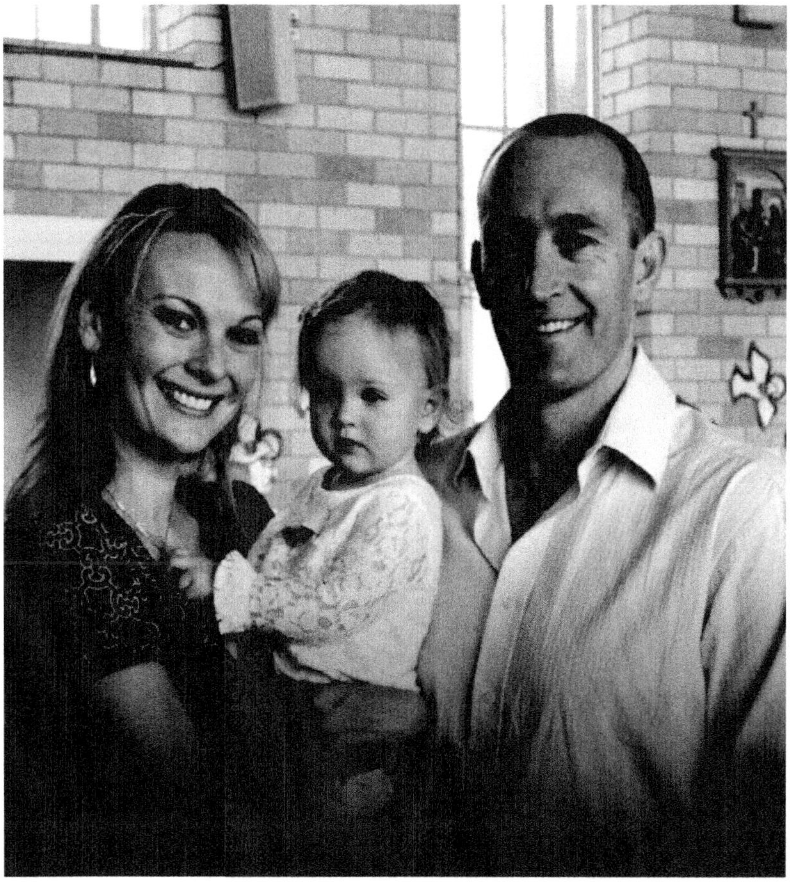

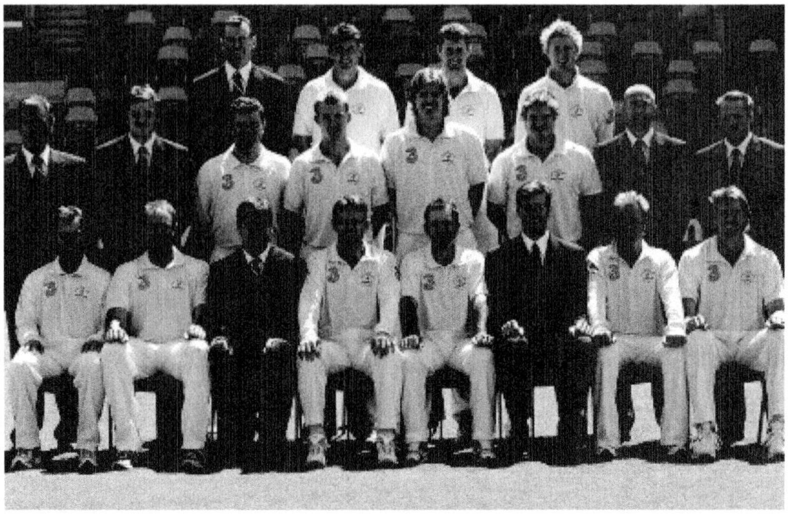

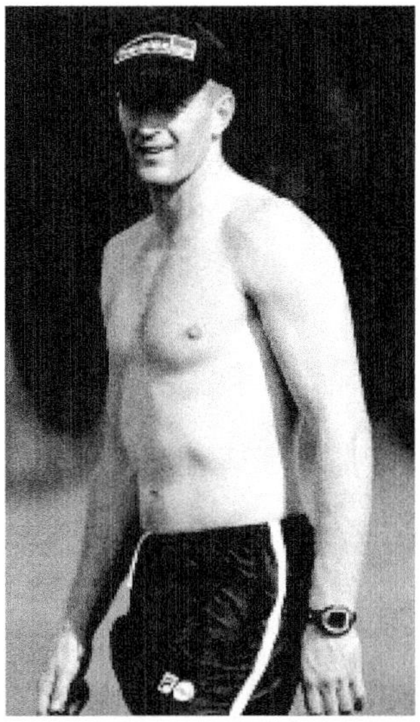

"I worked through my whole time with cancer, it was my coping strategy. In hindsight I should have taken a bit of time out to have a break."

"One incredibly positive thing I learnt from my time with cancer is the "Gratitude Exercise" where you sit down every week and write down five great things in your life at that time."

I wish people knew it was absolutely okay to talk openly to others and admit to them that you're scared.

April 15, 2008 is the day that life stood still for Andrew May, 38. It was the day he found out that a routine skin check and subsequent biopsy – that he had only at the insistence (nagging!) of his wife – had resulted in a life changing diagnosis. With just six weeks until the birth of their first child, Andrew had to go in for surgery to remove a malignant melanoma from the back of his left shoulder.

"Mostly we think of dealing with cancer as treating it, but what about trying to prevent it? Let's educate. We all have to teach our kids from a young age about what they can do to try and minimise cancer."

"A lot of people get through cancer and then go through this real dip afterwards. I've since learnt that it's called "Post Cancer Fatigue" and it definitely happened to me. I lost my mojo. I lost my spark."

LAUREN HEHIR

"Sometimes it's alright to stop fighting."

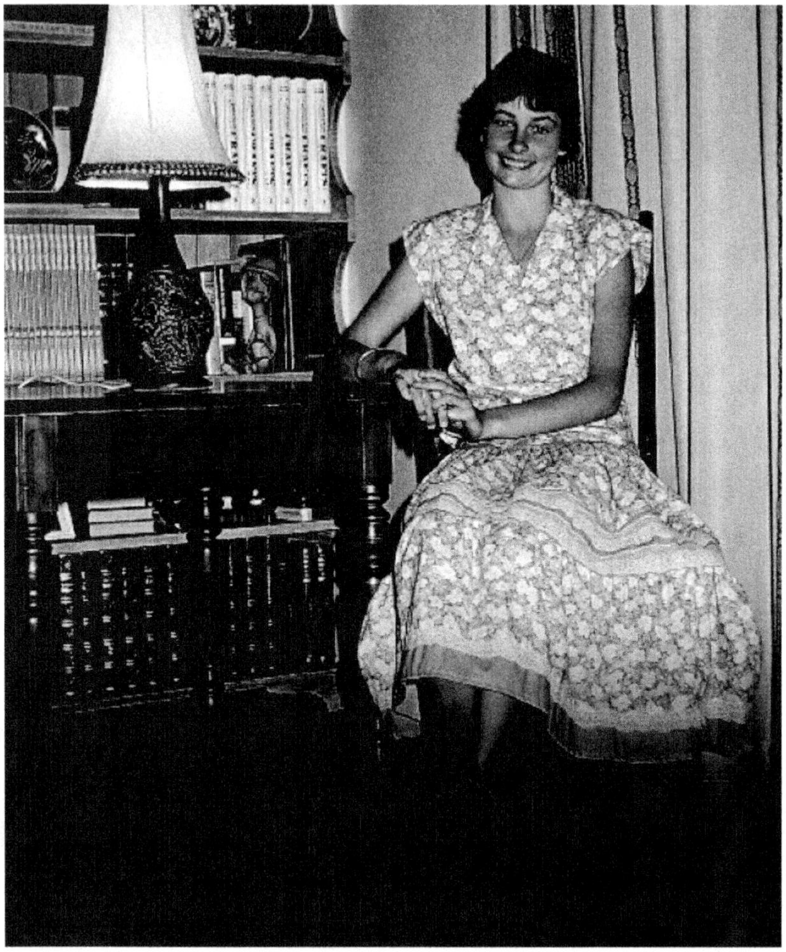

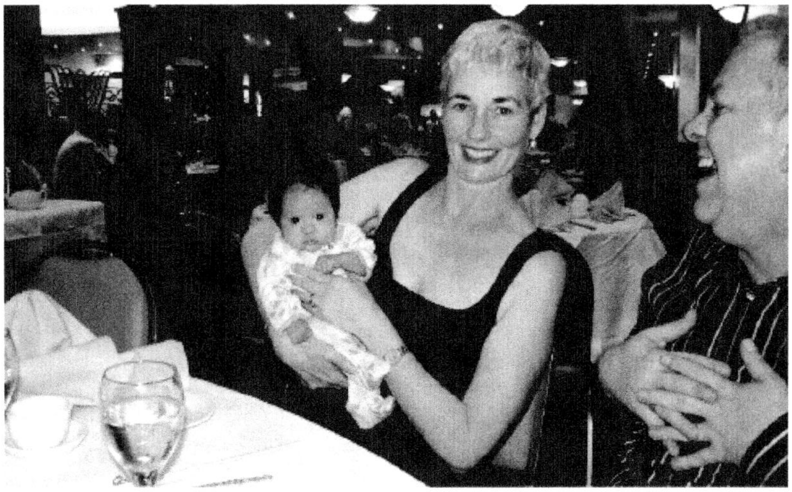

Palliative Care Nurse, Lauren Hehir, 46, once looked after a young boy who had multiple surgeries to save his life. He had his leg amputated below his knee, and his foot sewn on to the stump backwards to mimic a knee joint so that he would eventually be able to wear a below knee leg prosthesis. Through all this he just continued to try and 'be a kid'. Eventually the boy just couldn't do it anymore and gave up and, when he died, Lauren says she felt enormous relief for him and his family.

"Be honest with the patient, most of the time they know what's going on anyway."

Sometimes families want to keep the truth about a patient's illness from them. They say things like 'Please don't tell my daughter she has cancer – she doesn't know.' or 'Don't say the word hospice to my mother, just tell her it's a hospital.' Lauren says this just complicates things and often the patient – especially if they're a kid – is very intuitive and about their illness and deserves to know the truth.

"I can be self-centred at times; but working in palliative care gives my life perspective and helps me to stay grounded. As much as the patients need me, I also need them – it's a good balance."

Lauren remembers going to work one day feeling very down as her husband had recently lost his job. That morning a young mother had died and, as Lauren walked down the hallway to her office, she heard the woman's two-year-old boy start to cry. While it probably had nothing to do with the death it brought a new perspective to her own situation. She says 'I remember sitting down in my office and giving myself a stern lecture. I still had my family and my health – this child had lost his mother'.

STEPHANIE BUTLAND

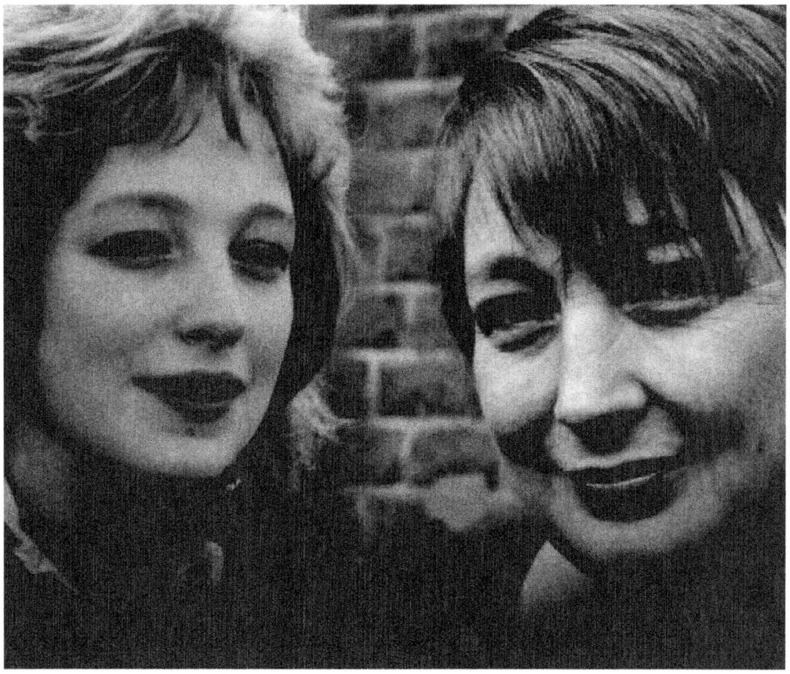

"Think very carefully about how you spend your time. Before diagnosis, as well as doing my job I was running a cake business and doing a psychology degree. The business and the degree went, because I realised I wasn't enjoying them. Now if I'm reading a book and not enjoying it by page 50, I stop. If I'm watching a play and I don't think it's any good, I leave at the interval."

For Stephanie Butland, 39, life was rolling along quite nicely before she found a lump in her breast (she was getting dressed for a night out and it was poking out of her bra and 'totally spoiling the line!'). Since her treatment she has moved 350 miles away from London to rural Northumberland, where life is quieter and calmer. She thinks she would never have contemplated this before, but now she says it feels like the most natural and exciting thing in the world.

"Recognise and accept when you need a bit of help before you get to the tantrums and tears stage. Remind yourself that you are surrounded by people who want to support you, even if sometimes you need to show them how."

Even though you have a cancer, life can still be good. And I mean properly good, not "good considering you've got cancer". While in treatment I had weekends away, long gossipy lunches, walks in beautiful places, and it was just as enjoyable, if not better, than it would have been before. A dance with cancer is not unremitting misery, it's just another stage in your life and, like all the other times, there's good and bad all mixed in together.

CLAUDETTE NEAVE

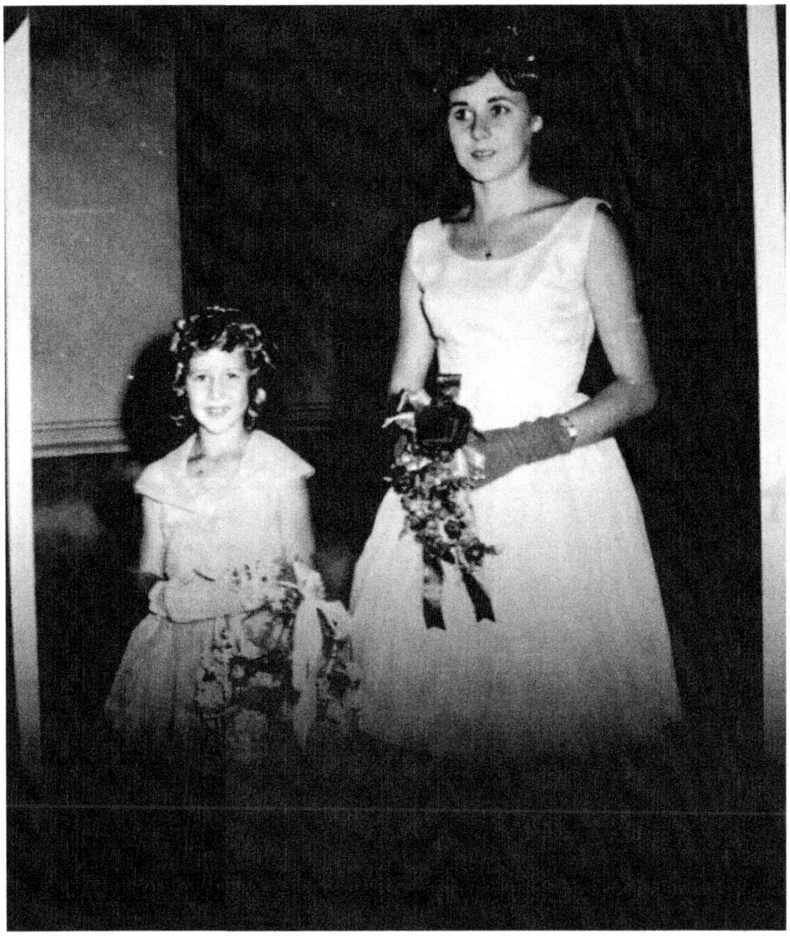

"You have to get a bit angry with cancer. You have to ask, "Hey! What the hell are you doing? Why am I going through this?" You can't stay in that anger though. You have to get angry and then let it go. Anger, acceptance, work through it and then move forward."

Claudette Neave's mother and grandmother both died of breast cancer, so she wasn't entirely surprised when she was diagnosed herself at 50 years of age. She had her breast removed and 'thought that would be that'. So it came as a shock when there was a recurrence of the cancer in the breast that wasn't there, right before she was about to have open-heart surgery in 2007. She underwent chemotherapy for the cancer and vowed to move on with her life. Not long after this, some recurring groin and hip pain saw her at the doctors again. This time she was told that she had metastatic bone cancer, as a secondary to the breast cancer. Now 65, she is currently in remission and says, 'I intend to be around for a long time yet.'

"It's really important to educate yourself. No-one told me that you can get a recurrence of cancer in exactly the same place. I wish the doctors had indicated to me that it was a possibility so it wasn't such a shock."

I always spoke to my kids about cancer because my mum and grandma died at such a young age. I didn't want them to be scared of it, but to know that it happens and you have to be careful of what you do and how you look after yourselves.

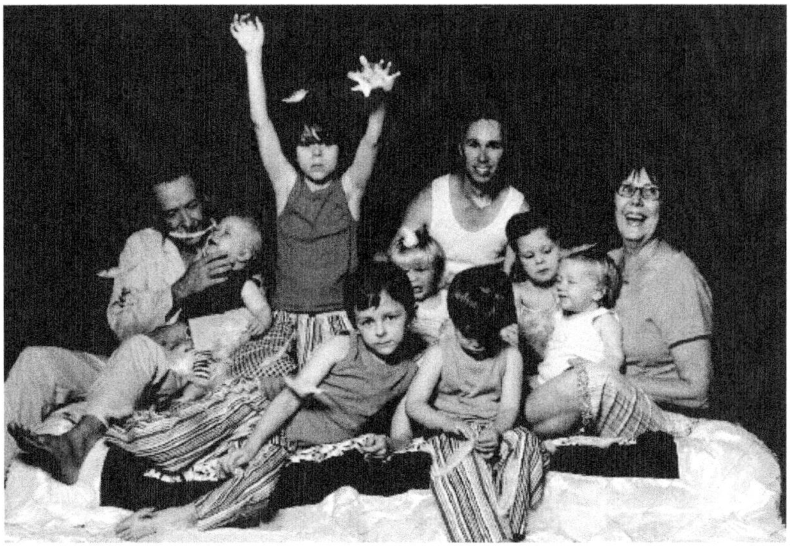

"You have to have faith, whether it be in a higher being or just in the people around you. I'm not overly religious, but I prayed and prayed to God and especially Mary McKillop, and I really believe that she led me to the kinesiologist that I've come to regard as "my healer"

TANYA CALDWELL-EYLES

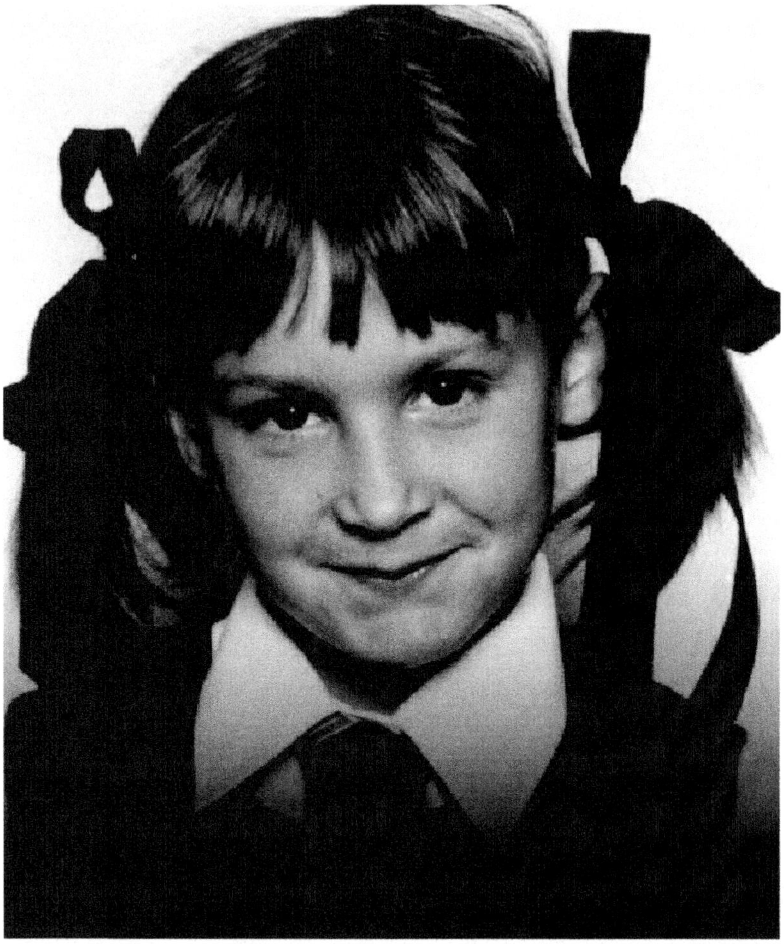

"Akin to childbirth and motherhood, the pain of cancer eventually subsides leaving behind a tiny miracle and a whole new perspective on life."

"I have learned that positive exists in every situation, but it can be a shy little creature, sometimes found trying to hide behind the generally larger one called pain. If we can just

find the strength to move positive to the front, we end up with positive pain. No matter how small it may seem at first, when we find the positive and focus on it, we gain the power to not just move on, but to evolve."

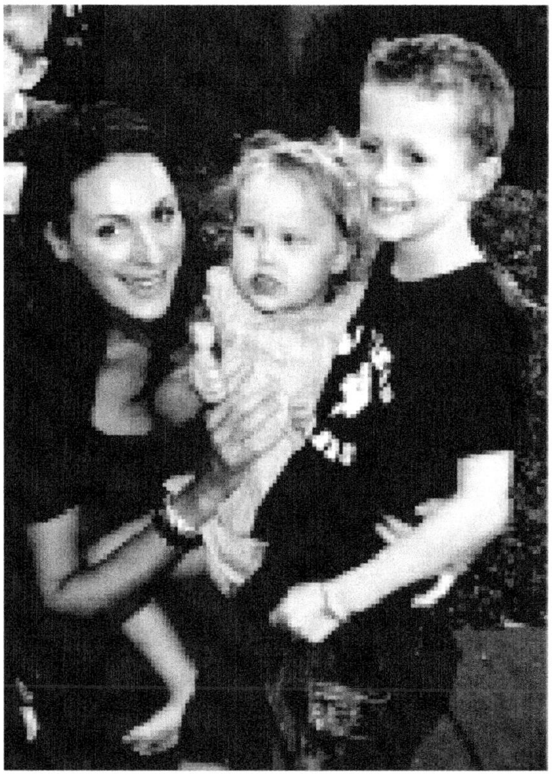

Tanya Caldwell-Eyles, 37, remembers watching her mother fight back tears as they left the hospital after visiting Tanya's grandmother who was dying of breast cancer. More vivid is Tanya's memory of her mother's words 'So much pain, so little dignity ... if I ever get that sick ... I just want to go ... life is about quality not quantity.' These words came back to haunt Tanya as she held her mother's hand when she too died from breast cancer years later. Then, when Tanya was

35, her own breast cancer journey began. In February 2009, she discovered that she carries the BRCA2 gene, in May 2009, Tanya was diagnosed with breast cancer. She says the 'benefit' of her younger experiences made an aggressive response to an aggressive disease easier. After undergoing a double mastectomy and reconstructive surgeries, she is the first in three generations of women to survive breast cancer.

JUSTIN PRATT

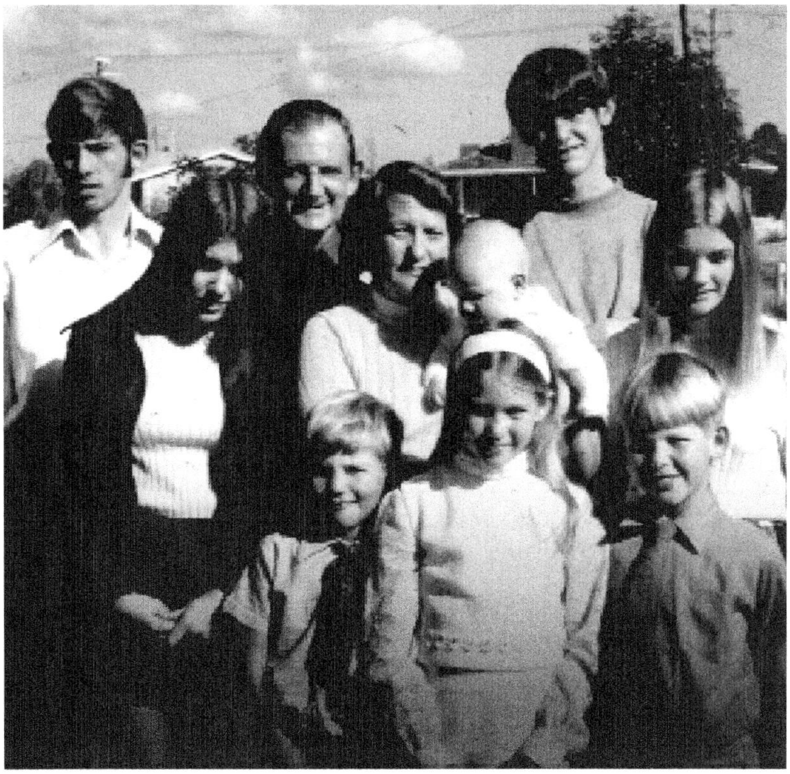

"What you do today has consequences far into the future. Sure quitting an addiction is a hard fight, but you have to compare that to the terrible battle you'll have to get through to survive the many horrific diseases that follow on from that addiction, and the devastating affect that will have on your family."

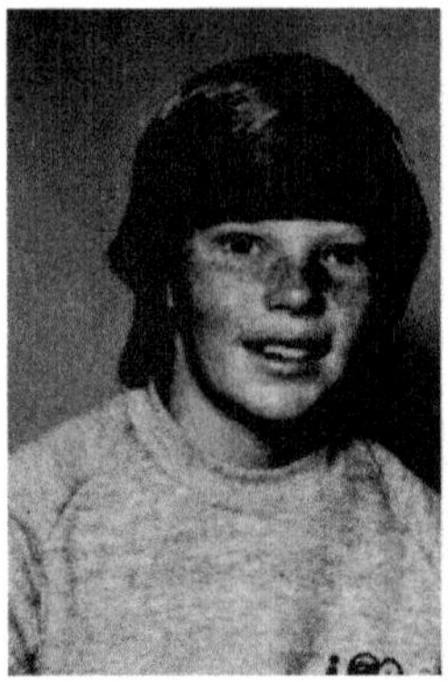 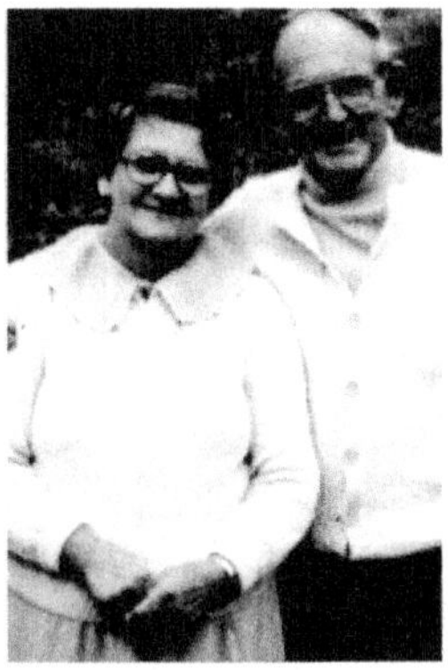 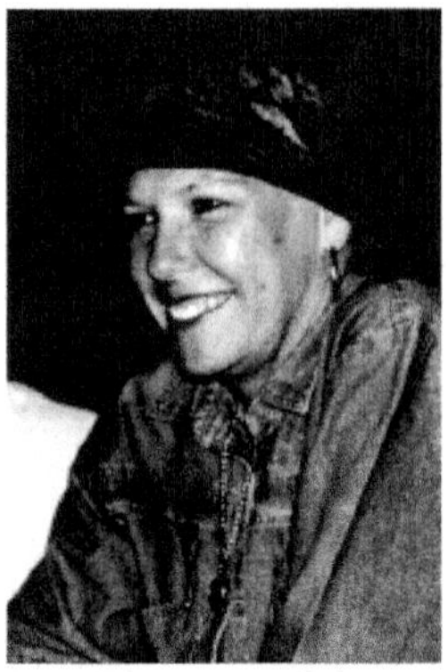

"So, for your children's sake, you have to teach them about all the things they can do, and the life choices they can make that will influence how their life progresses. Not smoking is a simple one that I reiterate over and over and over again."

When Justin Pratt was just 14 years old, his father passed away at age 64 from lung cancer, having smoked all his life. Now at 39, Justin is vehemently against smoking and is already ingraining the 'Don't smoke' message into his small children. Justin rides in the Tour de Cure in memory of his father, and also his sister who passed away from breast cancer in her early 40's.

BRONNIE TAYLOR

Clinical Nurse, consultant and McGrath Breast Care Nurse, Bronnie Taylor, 41, still remembers the first cancer patient she looked after until the end. When they met, the woman already had metastatic disease which was progressive and incurable, and Bronnie just loved working with her and her family because she was able to see how cancer allows people to prioritise and simplify their lives in such a powerful way.

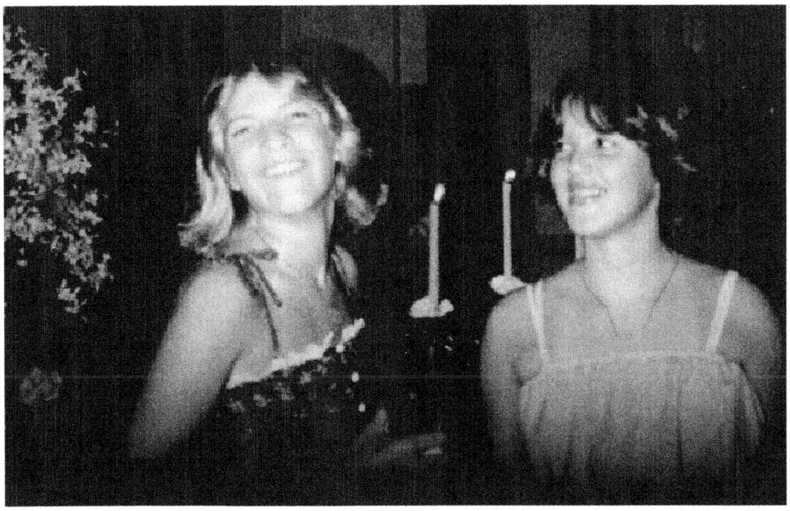

"We just take it as a given that we go on from day to day. When someone has been diagnosed with a life limiting illness it gives them that opportunity to say, "You know what, I'm going to really do what's important and I'm going to make life simpler." There's lot to be said for a simple life and I think after a cancer diagnosis it almost empowers you to do that."

"Cancer is a much more positive story than it ever used to be. Our treatment is so much better, survival rates are much higher, many people even continue to work full time throughout their treatment."

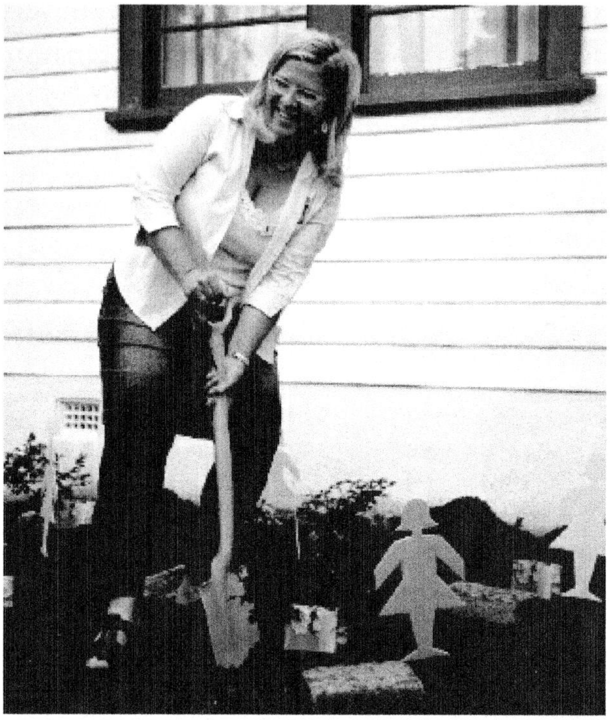

The key to getting through it is seeing what suits you and doing it your way. There's no right or wrong way to do cancer.

Seven years ago Bronnie's brother-in-law developed leukaemia which required a stem cell transplant from a donor they eventually found in Sweden. Bronnie says that, while she always tries to be empathetic and look after people as she would care for one of her own loved ones, this gave her an incredibly valuable insight into being on the other side of treatment.

ROBYN CANNA

"Hospitals are like a shopping centre with a revolving door. Fantastic places, wonderful doctors, but sometimes you've got to stop the escalator and stand your ground. You must be vigilant about everything, you must listen to everybody and you must ask questions."

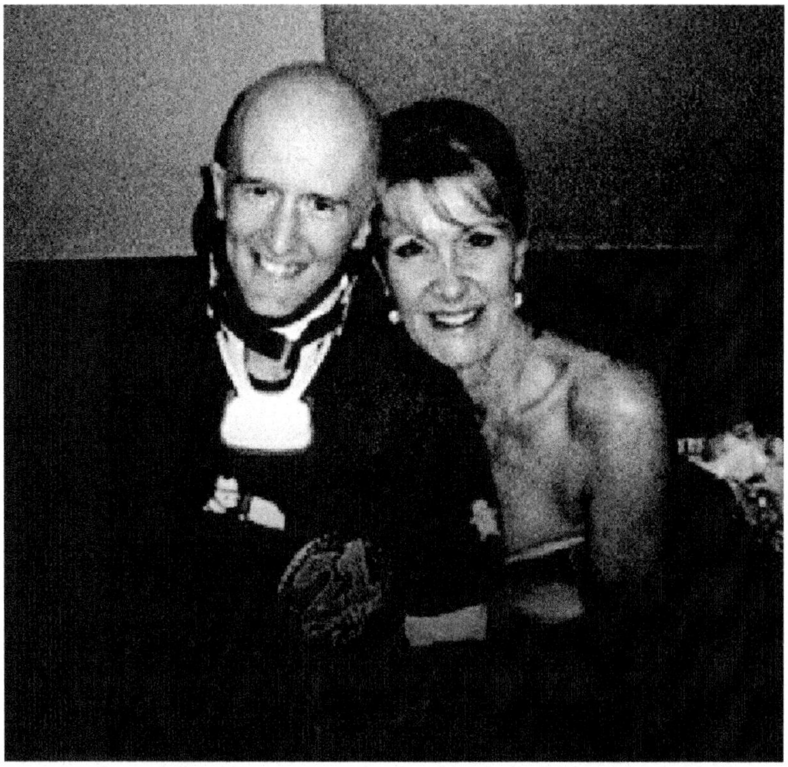

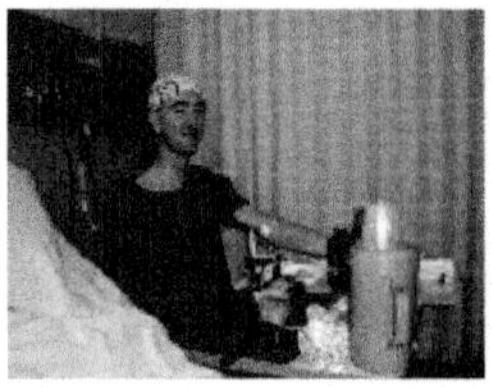

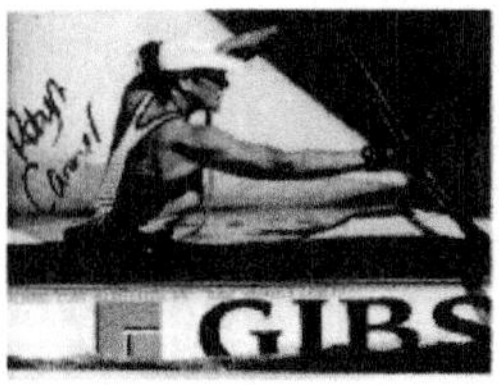

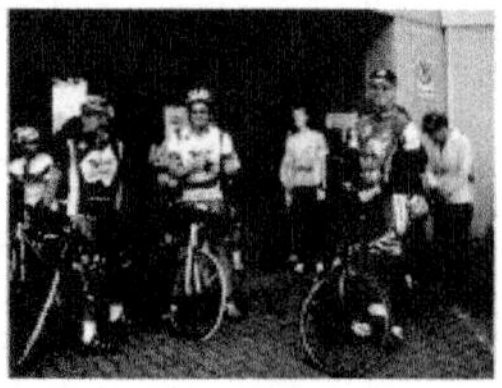

"Be vigilant. This gives your child a sense of emotional security that someone has their back. Their doctors have their body, but who has their back? The parent."

"It is of utmost importance to know everything about your body, what it's going through and more to the point, what you're doing with it because everything has a side effect."

At the age of 36, Robyn Canna went for a routine pap smear where they picked up the early stages of cervical cancer. She was fortunate to have all the cancer removed and has been in remission for the past 18 years. However, now, she is caring for her son Scott, 22 who is currently living with non-Hodgkin's lymphoma.

Once a year I have a full body scan. Some will say, "Oh, radiation causes cancer." But cancer that you've already got can kill you if you don't know it's there. And it's very good at hiding.

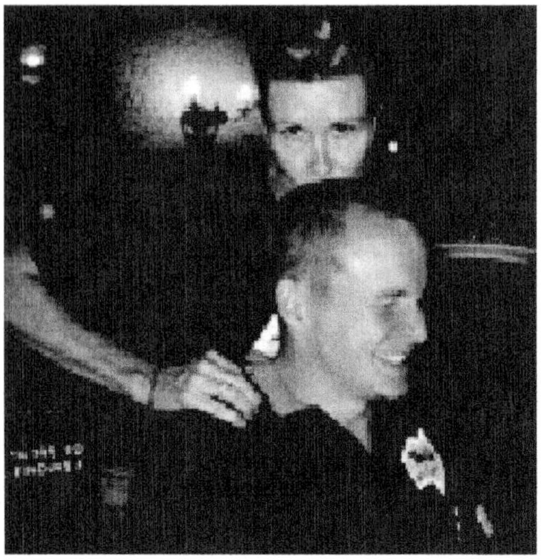

MICHAEL MILTON

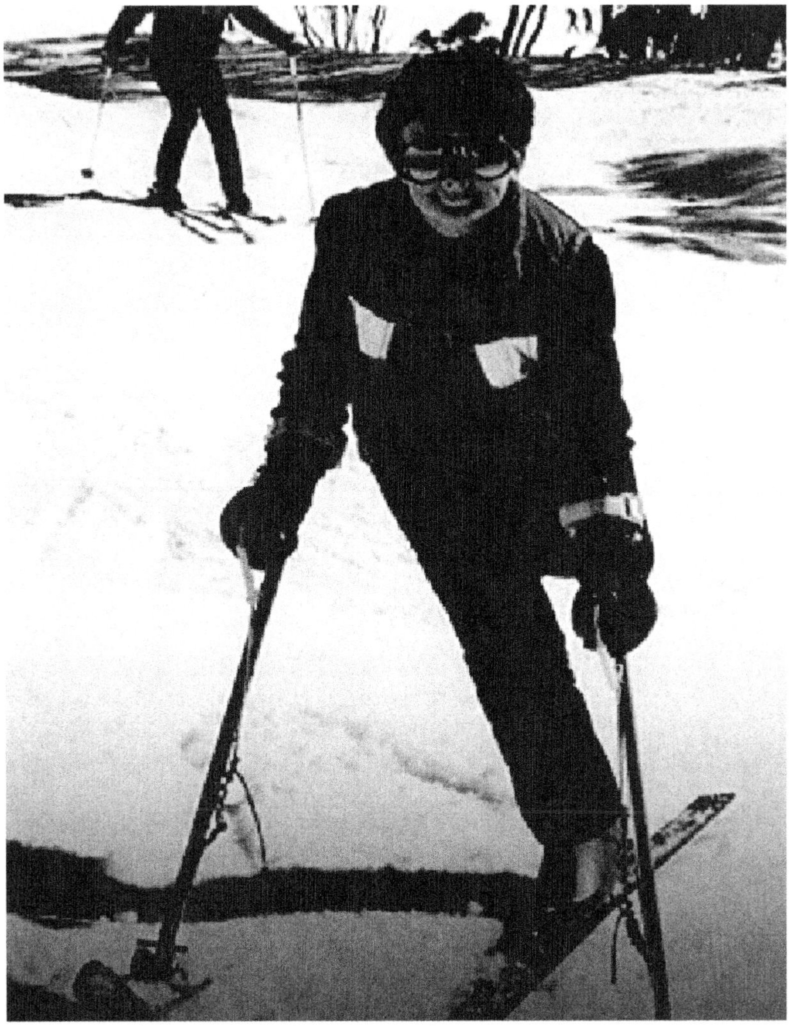

"Being an amputee is a relatively small deal compared to a cancer diagnosis. You're talking about a leg versus your life. When you think about what is important in life, it's being healthy and happy, having something you love to do, a wonderful family and a great group of supportive

friends. Compared to that, only having one leg has bugger all to do with anything really."

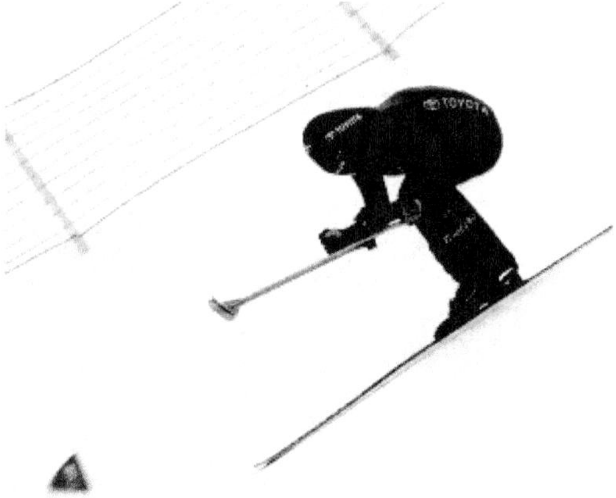

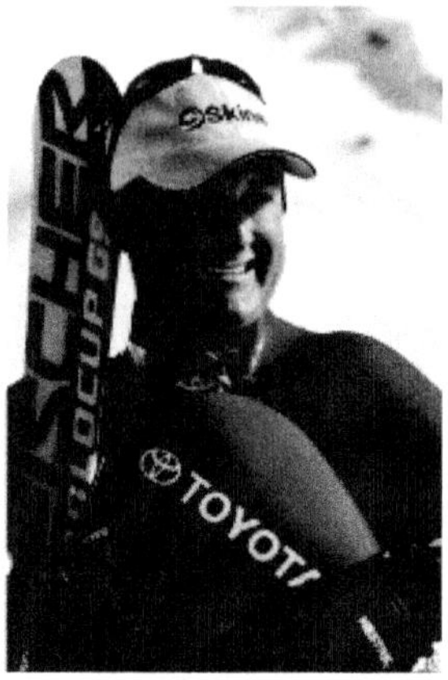

"When I see a kid in a similar situation, I feel more for the parents than the child, because in some ways the kid is protected by their naivety. But the parents and other adults are the ones that the diagnosis hits the hardest."

"It's very natural for your paternal instincts to kick in and want to protect your child from any further harm for the rest of their lives, but that can actually have an extremely negative effect on them, because you don't let them go out and do things that normal kids do; all the things that are required as part of learning and becoming a balanced human being."

At age nine, Michael Milton was diagnosed with an osteogenic sarcoma in his left leg, which resulted in 18 months of chemotherapy and having his leg amputated above the knee. But this didn't deter

Michael away from his dream – skiing. He went on to win 11 world championship medals, including six gold, and 11 Olympic medals, also including six gold. More recently, he took up track cycling and was loving it and achieving great results when, in June 2007, his life was again interrupted with a bout of cancer, this time oesophageal. He underwent chemotherapy, radiotherapy and surgery to remove his oesophagus and two-thirds of his stomach. Amazingly, Michael, now aged 37, not only recovered, he went on to qualify for the cycling team at the Beijing games.

SUE MELIA

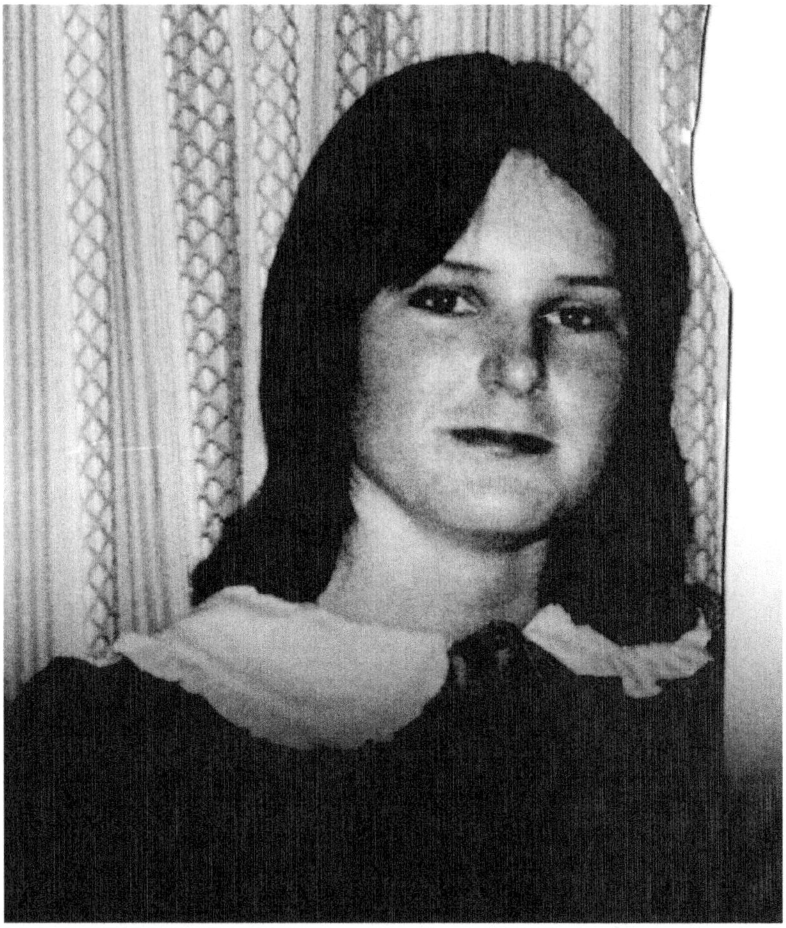

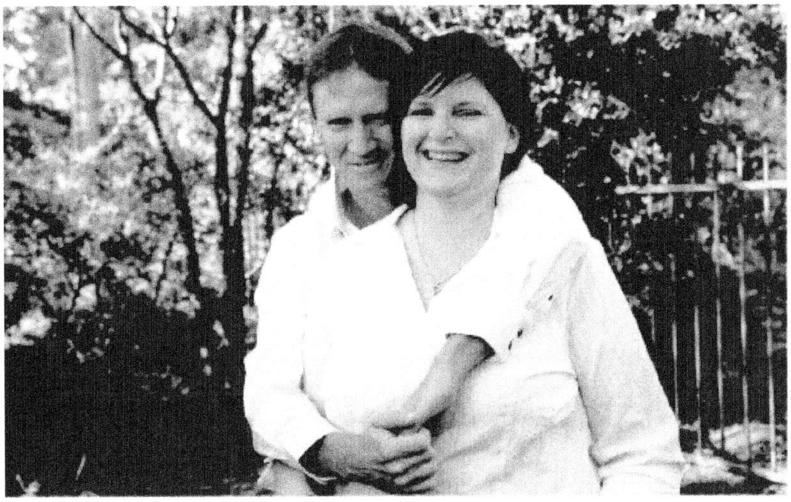

"If you're having any types of abnormal symptoms you should keep a diary of them, and if they go on for any longer than three or four weeks you must go and see a doctor."

Sue Melia, now 45, understands why ovarian cancer is called 'the silent killer' because she put her symptoms – bloating, menstrual changes and being more tired than usual – down to regular variations in her cycle or a slowing metabolism due to age. She went to the doctor and, after some initial scans, was referred quickly to a Gynaecological Oncologist who opened up his surgery on a Saturday to see her. Sue says, 'When a specialist sees you on the weekend, you know you're in trouble'. She was diagnosed with ovarian cancer and had surgery three days later. Sue has three teenage daughters and recently attended her oldest daughter graduation from high school, one of the many things she thought she might never see.

"Don't let anyone take away your hope."

Sue had been suffering from depression for a couple of years before her diagnosis with ovarian cancer. She now has a hunch the cancer growing inside her might have been part of the cause. One of her doctors said, 'Now, with your history of depression, how do I know that you're going to finish this treatment?'

Sue looked him straight in the eye and said, 'Excuse me, I have a husband and three teenage daughters, I promise you I WILL finish this'. Sue says that in her darkest days with depression she actually thought life was just too hard and that 'even cancer would be better than this!' Now, after getting through her cancer and in remission she is the happiest she's been in years and lives in hope for a long life surrounded by her family and friends.

HELEN MUNROE

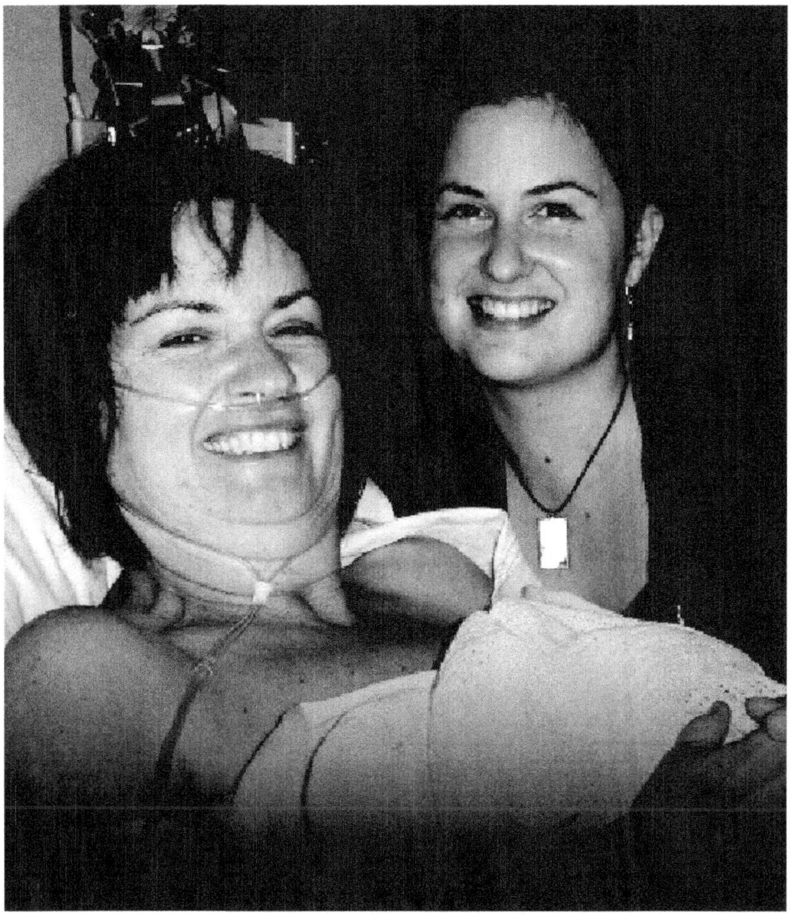

"I think you have to trust your doctors. I wasn't one of these people that got on the net and started researching alternative things, I figured they are the specialists so the information they have had to be far greater and more up to date than any internet site I was going to stumble upon."

"I tried a support group for a while, and while it was fun and I met some really nice people, the conversation was all too often about cancer. I guess I just wanted to forget about it. Been there, done that, move on."

"Share your experience with your friends and family, and it doesn't feel so bad."

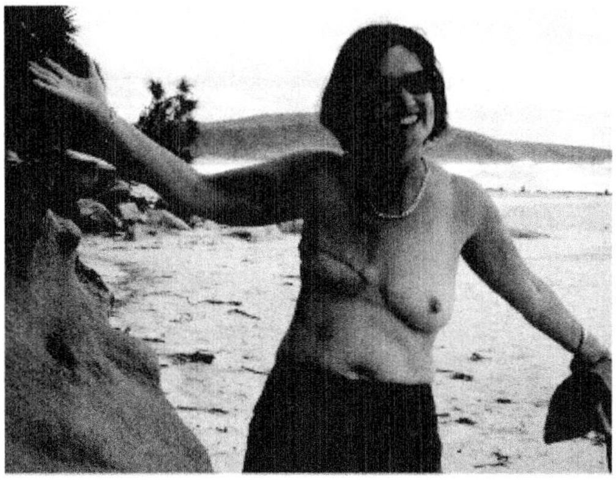

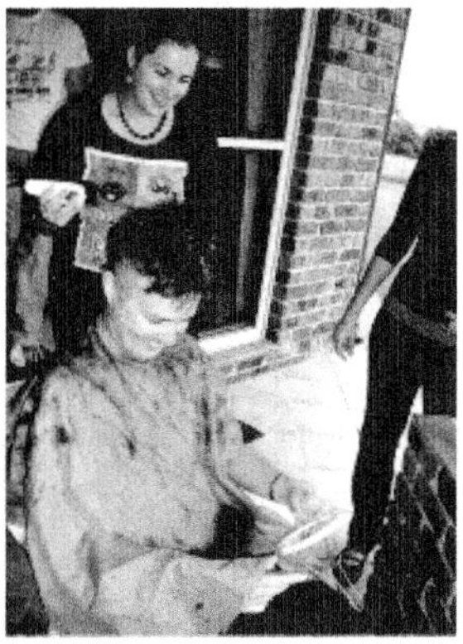

"I told friends, "Treat me like you always have. Don't be overly kind to me, because I will begin to think I'm going to die." I look back on it now as a real party year! One of the best years of my life."

While Helen Munroe, 53, was undergoing treatment for breast cancer in 2007, she decided to photograph the whole process and share it with her friends who lived locally, and her two children who live in Sydney. She was accompanied by at least one girlfriend to every doctor's appointment and her daughter, Hannah, flew home to be there for all the important things like her lumpectomy, plastic moulding of her real breast before surgery, her mastectomy, and – of course – giving mum an awesome mohawk. Once, fairly soon after her mastectomy, Helen was at a fairly isolated beach with a girlfriend, and they decided to take a few topless photos. Her newsletter to friends and family the next day said, 'I went to the beach yesterday. No whales, no dolphins, just the one white pointer.'

PROFESSOR JOHN RASKO

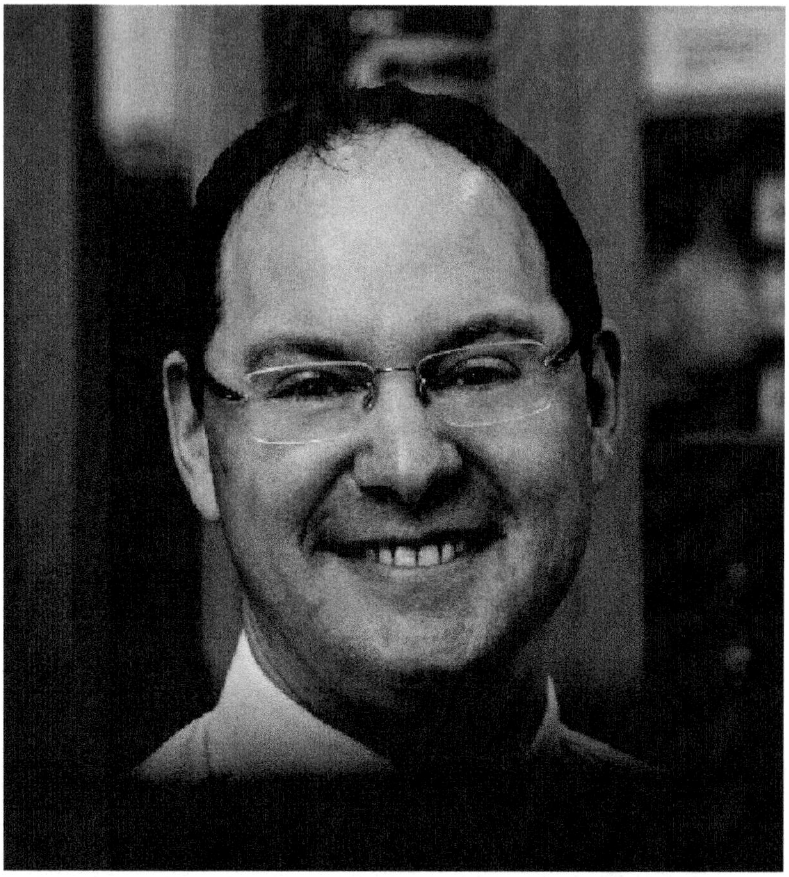

"People should be aware that government funding in Australia is woefully inadequate to translate new therapies and new discoveries that will ultimately assist people suffering from cancer. As a nation, we can do much better for those in need."

"Important discoveries in medical research can make an enormous difference to the lives of

those hit by cancer. A new therapy based on solid biomedical research not only improves the immediate wellbeing of those individuals right now, but it also changes the path for everyone suffering from that disease in the future. In this way, we strive for continuous improvements in cancer care and seek to bring hope to families during difficult times."

"When I was training there were diseases that were almost a death sentence, but are now curable. Consider the blood cancer called acute lymphoblastic leukaemia. In the past, about 90 percent of children under the age of five who had this diagnosis would die within a few years. Now, that statistic is reversed so that nearly 90 percent are likely to experience some form of cure from modern therapies. Other cancers like chronic myeloid leukaemia, testicular cancer and certain types of lymphoma have provided examples where medical research has revolutionised outcomes."

Professor John Rasko, 49, is Head of the Department of Cell and Molecular Therapies at Royal Prince Alfred Hospital; Head of the Gene and Stem Cell Therapy Program at the Centenary Institute of Cancer Medicine; and Professor of Medicine at the University of Sydney. He is a world-renowned gene therapy and stem cell scientist and practising haematologist whose research has been successful in uncovering new mechanisms of leukaemia, understanding blood hormones, identifying the genetic causes of kidney diseases and clinical trials of new biological therapies for cancer and bleeding disorders.

"Everyone needs to know that smoking promotes most forms of cancer. Often people are shocked to hear that smoking also increases voice-box cancer, kidney cancer, leukaemia and so on. Smoking produces horrible toxins and allows many dozens of cancer causing chemicals to enter the bloodstream through the smoke. These poisons damage DNA and lead to cancer causing mutations. Try and prevent the cancer forming by stopping smoking yourself or convincing your loved ones to stop. The new patches and drugs to assist can be really helpful."

ALI BROINOWSKI

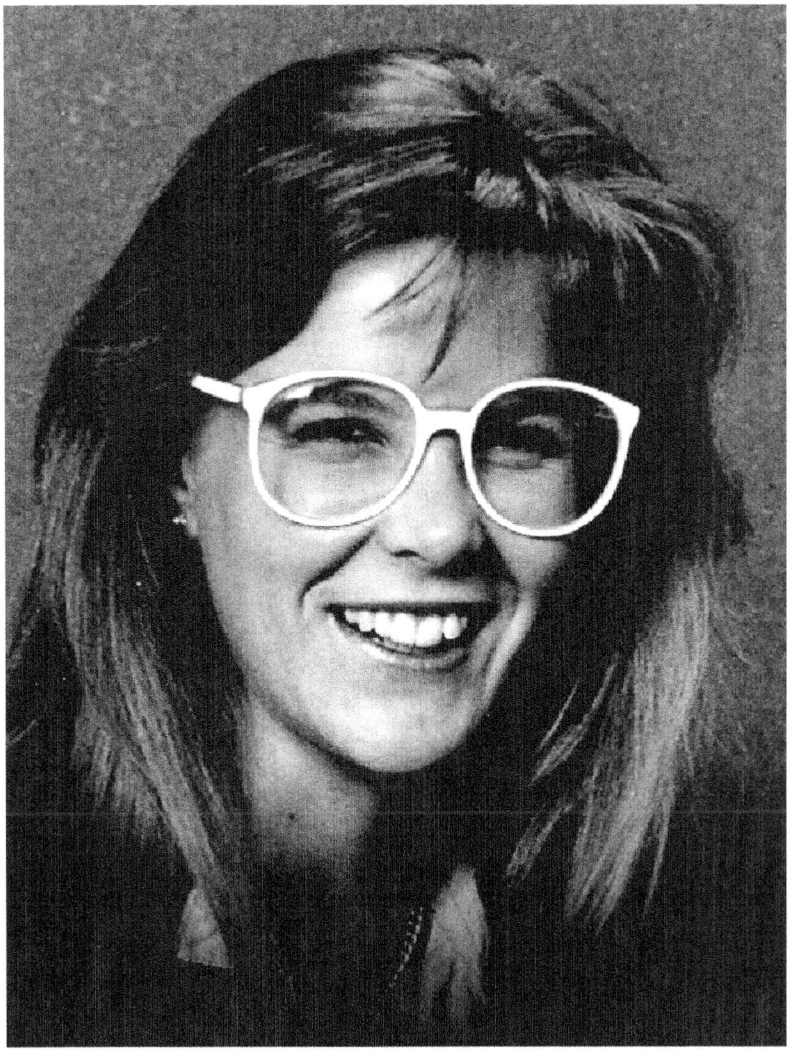

"Cancer was one of the best things that ever happened to me, it changed the way I live. Before having it I was just bumbling along living paycheck to paycheck, weekend to weekend, holiday to holiday – without any plans or goals

or conscious decisions about life. Very self-centered and all about me."

When Ali Broinowski, 42 was seven months pregnant with her second child she rolled over in bed and noticed her right breast was sore. By six o'clock that night the lump was the size of a golf ball but Ali couldn't have it seen to straight away as she had to attend the funeral of her sister in law who had died that day from bowel cancer. Within a week Ali had been diagnosed with aggressive breast cancer and had one mastectomy at seven months pregnant, a caesarian three weeks later followed by chemo while still in the maternity ward. She then had a second mastectomy and breast reconstruction after the three months of chemotherapy were over.

"Now I do things because I want to do them not because I should, or because other people want me to."

"I went to my underwear drawer and got rid of all the ugly, practical underwear, the really hideous stuff. I said to myself "I'm never going to wear that shit again."

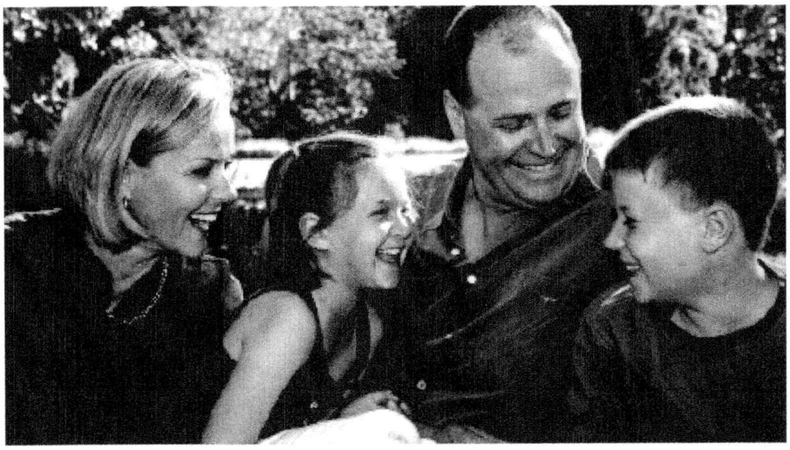

"You've got to get your head right. A friend was having chemo and the doctors told her that she needed to drink three to four litres of water a day to flush the poisons out of your body, and she'd be lucky to have two glasses of water because she felt so defeated. And she died. I'm not saying positivity is some "magic guarantee" of survival, but if you don't get your head right, you're not going to do all the things you simply must do to get better."

"The disease also taught me that I didn't need all the hanger-on friends. I had a big pruning process and let go the fifty million acquaintances it was fashionable to have, and focused on the friendships that I really cherished."

JULIET O'BRIEN

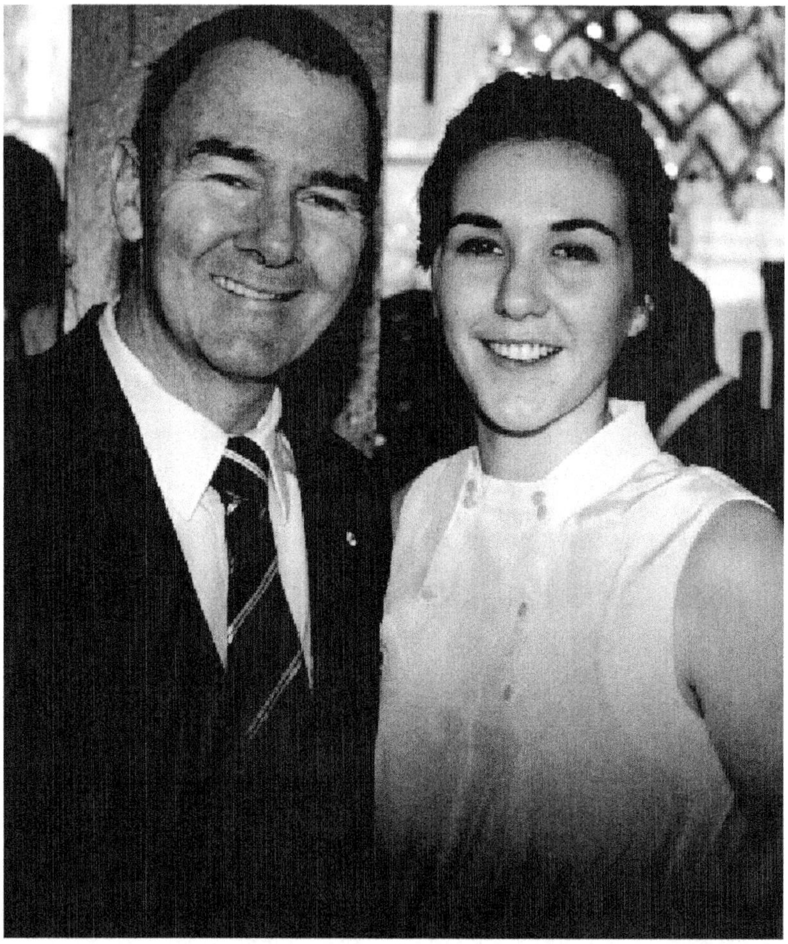

"Even though I've gone through it myself, I don't feel much wiser about what to tell people in a similar situation. One thing I would say is that you can't look too far ahead. Keep focussing on the moment."

"People who haven't had a parent go through cancer need to recognise that for them, life is

kind of suspended. It's like a hiatus and, from the day of the diagnosis, everything changes forever."

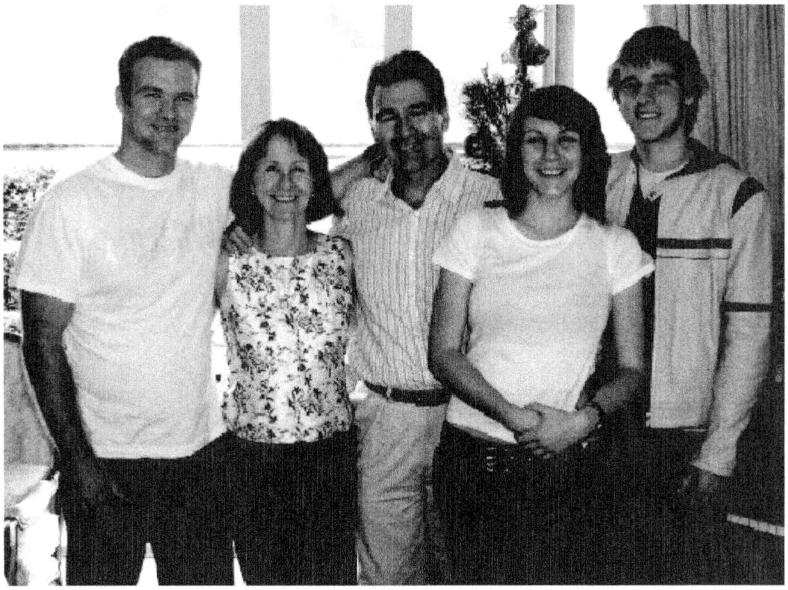

"You're trying to stay positive, because you want to believe he's got all the time in the world, but you have to balance that with the reality that he will probably die. You want to spend what time is left, together."

Juliet O'Brien, 26, is the daughter of renowned head and neck surgeon, Dr Chris O'Brien. Her father believed that cancer had to be fought aggressively, and as such, requested Dr Charlie Teo perform radical surgery on his brain. He went on to have five craniotomies, but eventually died from brain cancer in 2009.

"One thing dad always said was, "You need to bask in loads of love."

JO LOVELOCK

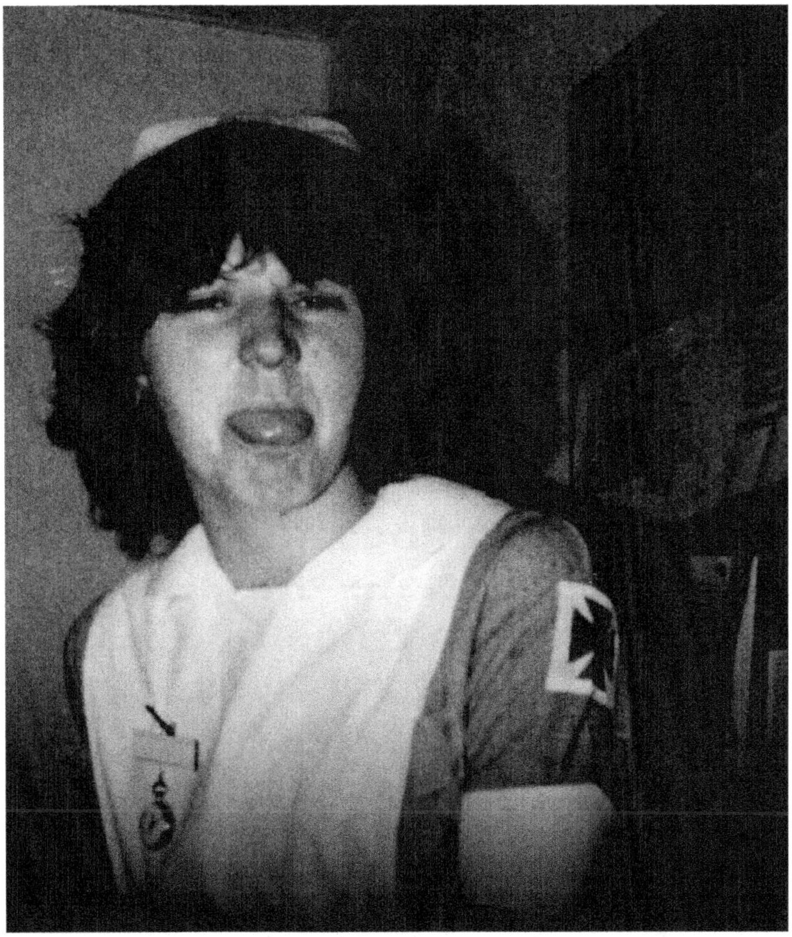

Cancer seems to permeate every part of your being when you're undergoing treatment, but you don't want your whole life to be cancer. You have to remind people that you're still you. I had to say, "Please treat me as 'Jo with a disease' not 'a disease called Jo.'"

While in the middle of chemo for breast cancer, Midwife Jo Lovelock, 52, was going for a blood test at the hospital where she worked when she bumped into a staff member who was known to whinge a bit. When the person predictably blurted out that she was 'having a bad hair day, whine, whine, whine etc,' Jo pulled a clump of hair out from the back of her head and barked 'YOU'RE HAVING A BAD HAIR DAY!' The woman screamed and ran off as Jo fell about laughing. Jo has gone on to become a Breast Care Nurse and help other women with breast cancer at their time of surgery.

"Keep your friends close and don't waste energy on those people or things that don't make you smile. Just politely delete the people from your phonebook that aren't helpful. But don't get upset by peoples' reaction to your cancer, they're just scared."

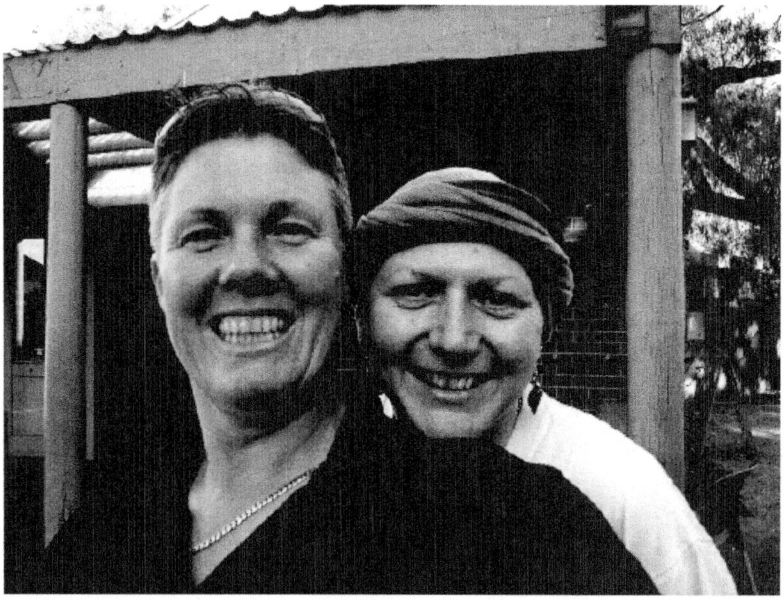

"Everyone is unique and your experience is that – just yours. Listen to people's views, smile then do whatever you want. Trust yourself and do lots of stuff you like."

"Accept that life is finite, and we can all make a difference to the world in small ways."

MEGAN GEORGE

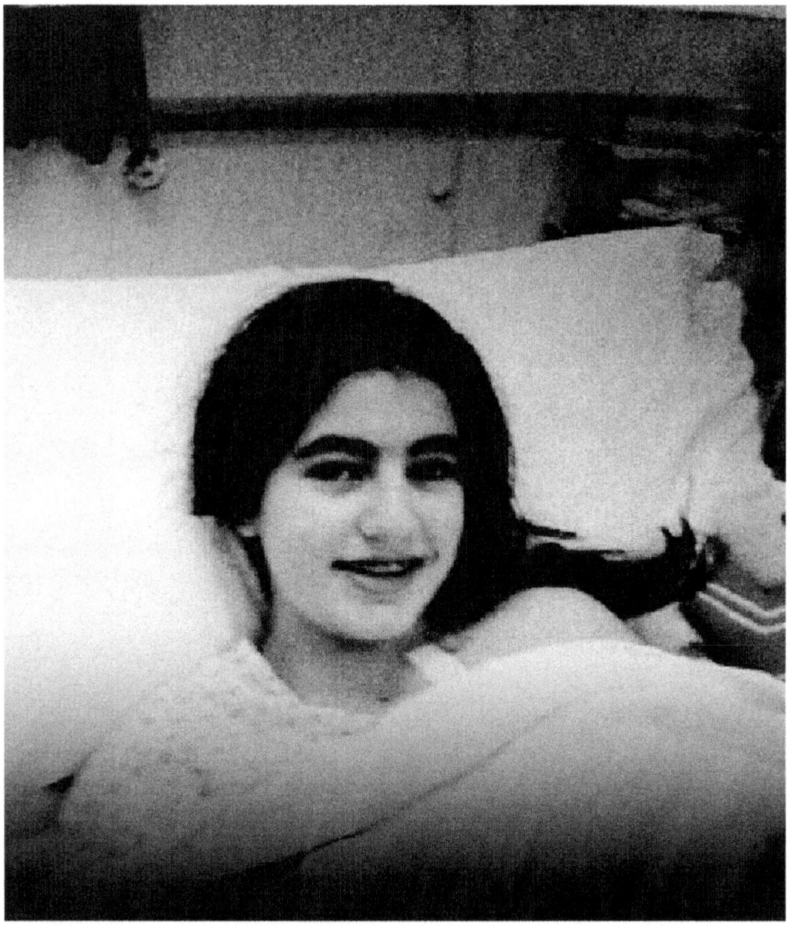

"A couple of small but practical tips – during chemo, go for the tonic water and fresh air to keep cool, both these things helped my nausea a lot. When you're having radiation keep some vitamin E cream and aloe vera around because your skin burns and needs a lot of soothing."

"I would tell parents of children with cancer to try and keep a smile on your face while you're around your child. Whenever I saw my Mum or Dad cry I would just assume I was going to die because I'd never see my parents cry, ever. I know it's the hardest thing in the world to do, but if you can keep a smile on your face it will really help your child's confidence and outlook on their disease."

In 2004, when she was only 12-years-old, Megan George discovered a lump on her collar bone and saw her GP. They did lots of tests, but didn't discover anything. A few months later another lump grew, and further tests revealed she had Hodgkin's lymphoma. She went through 24 months of chemo and radiation, missed two years of school, and still suffers from pains due to the myelin in her nerves being burnt off. She was contacted by the Make a Wish foundation and told them that her wish was to meet the Pope, so that's exactly what they made happen.

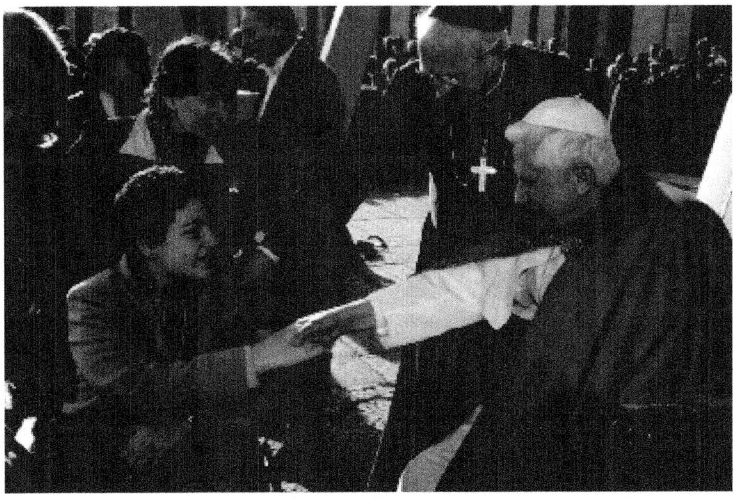

"Don't waste time asking "Why is this happening to me?" or whinging that "This isn't fair." I did an awful lot of that and one day just looked around my hospital ward and thought "Is it fair for anyone else in here? There are little babies in here, they haven't done anything that deserves cancer." None of it is fair."

Now when Megan feels any nausea or an upset stomach, she forgets all about it by talking to herself in a voice that sounds like Crocodile Dundee saying 'That ain't nausea, *chemo* is nausea.'

"I think if I could give myself advice it would be to just move forward and not to dwell on why?"

ROSEMARY PAUL

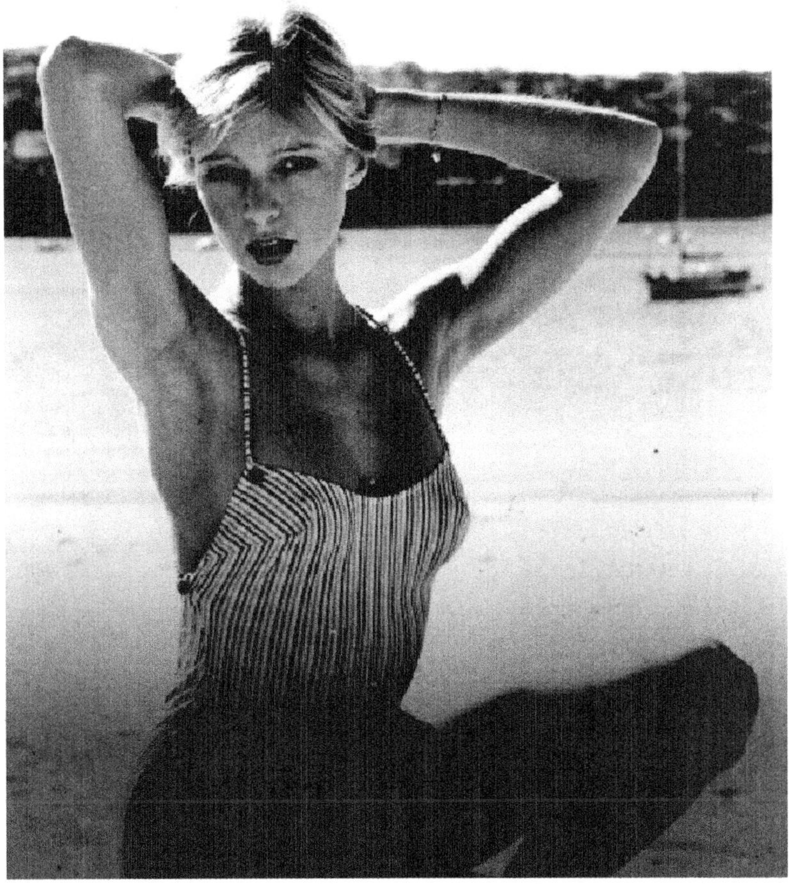

"The difference between me, or anybody who's been diagnosed with cancer, and the rest of population is that we know we're mortal. It's not like cutting your hair and letting it grow back again, once you've looked your mortality in the face, it feels like you're on a different train track to everybody else and you can't go back."

"Cancer strips away all your illusions of control. It tears away that facade that we all have where we think we are in charge. Ironically, once this happens, you can actually start concentrating on the things that really are under your control, which is a much healthier way to live."

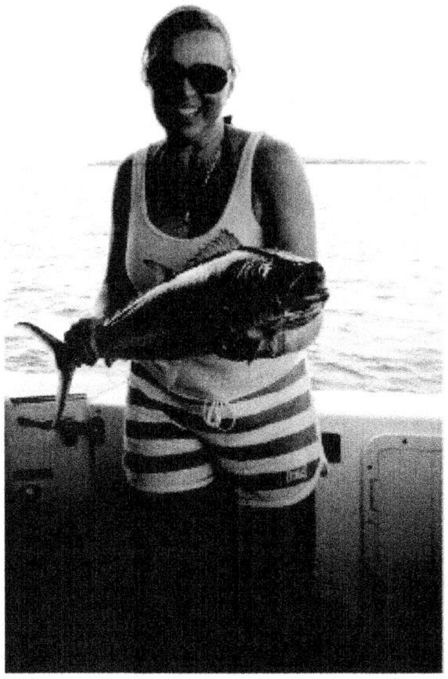

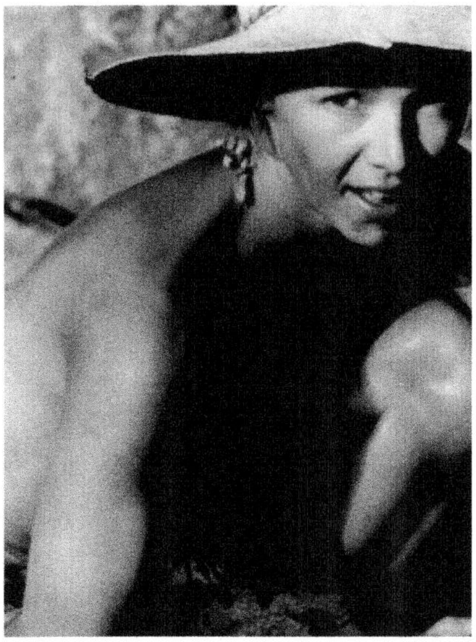

"I dislike the word survivor because I'm not surviving, I'm living. I'm living with the aftermath of being diagnosed and treated for cancer."

Rosemary Paul, 53, is a lymphoedema therapist who also regularly talks to cancer patients about her experiences with breast cancer 12 years ago. As it was on her bucket list, Rosemary did a comedy workshop and wrote a stand up routine about having had breast cancer, which she performed in front of all her family and friends. She talked openly about everything, even how a prosthesis and a summer singlet can leave you looking a bit asymmetrical when you're in the Woolies cold food section. (The women all laughed at this straight away, the men got it about sixty seconds later.) Her routine went so well that even her teenage kids – who promised they'd laugh even if she was terrible – said they loved it.

"Approach treatment for cancer the same way you'd approach buying a car or a house – you won't be told you've got cancer and then die ten minutes later. Even if doctors want to start treatment in two days time, that two days can be a space for taking some time, asking loads of questions, getting lots of advice, then making a logical, informed decision – not a quick panicky one."

SAM CAWTHORN

"If someone you are close to has cancer, continue to love them and treat them like you always have. Yes, they are going through a really tough time but they're still the same human being."

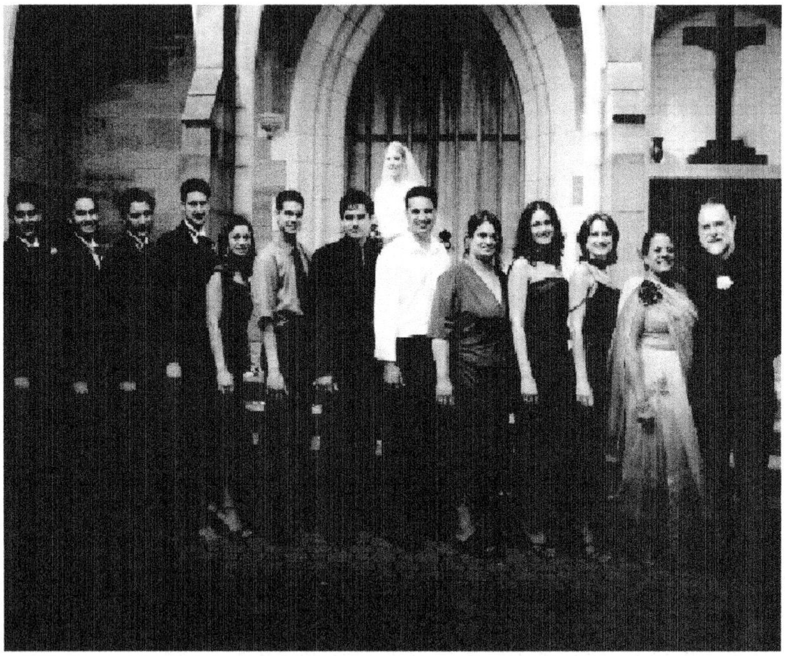

"A lot of us are scared of the questions, "What happens when you die? How do we pick ourselves up from this? Where is the hope after death?" If you know you're going to have to face those questions, talk about it beforehand – even with the person dying – and then you won't suddenly be in the deep end, with no idea how to swim."

"In hindsight, the best thing I did for my brother was just continue on with our relationship. I didn't try to be someone different, or tread lightly around him. We still messed about, I joked with him, teased him about his bald head, because he still wanted a mate. David didn't want someone to come around and feel sorry for him. He just wanted to be accepted as a normal person."

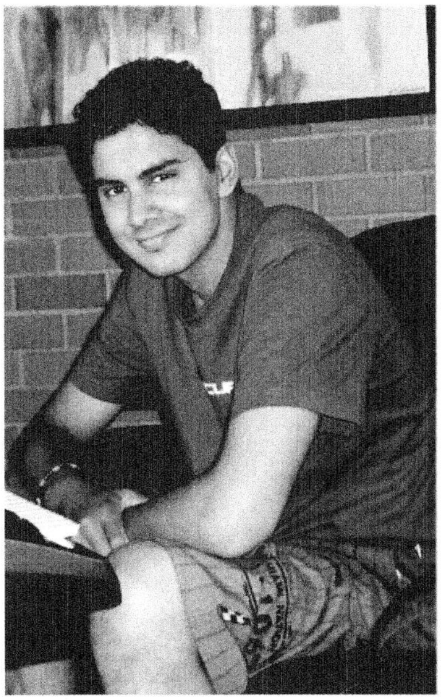
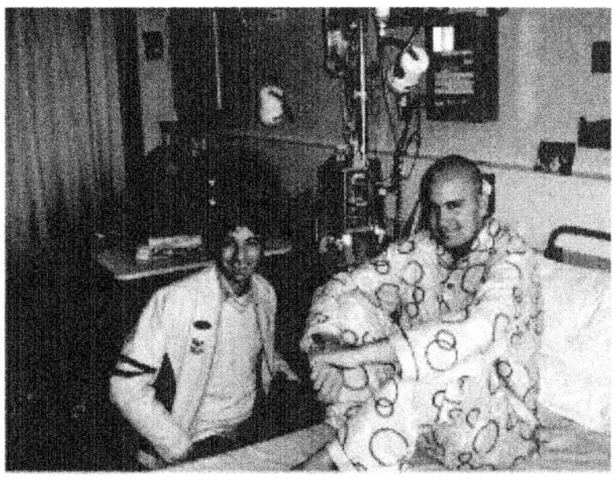
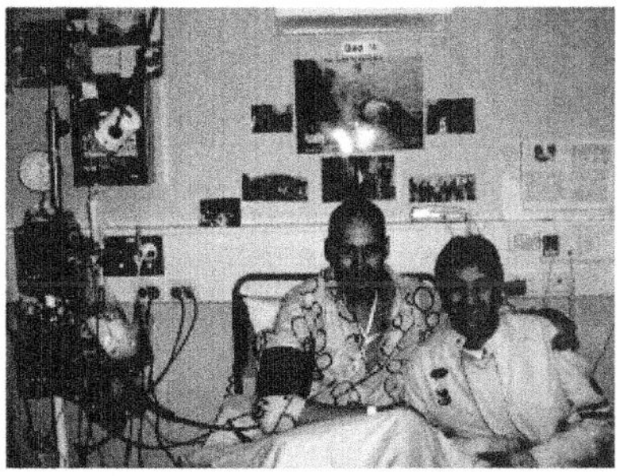

Sam Cawthorn, 31, grew up in a family of seven boys and four girls, and David – the youngest boy and Sam's best mate – was diagnosed with leukaemia just before he turned 20. David was in and out of hospital for around two years, then Sam stepped up to donate his bone marrow for a transplant. This kept the cancer at bay for a while, but after a year and a half there was nothing left they could do and David was given six weeks to live. Three weeks into that time Sam interviewed him on camera for an hour and a half, chatting away about his life story, his legacy and whether he was scared of dying. In hindsight, Sam says he somehow always thought David was going to make it, but he died about five weeks after the interview. The whole family watched the interview together two days after David passed away. Sam says, 'I still talk about David every single week without fail. When I think of him it's just like a person you haven't seen for a while, you still think of him, you still love him, you're still wondering what's going on in their life. So in a really great way he is completely alive in my heart.'

CORA ZILLICH

"As soon as I was diagnosed, I wanted to learn about my cancer – and cancer in general – in order to try to understand the enemy which had invaded my body. I knew then I'd be able to fight it better with the right nutrition, the right treatment, the right behaviour and the right fitness."

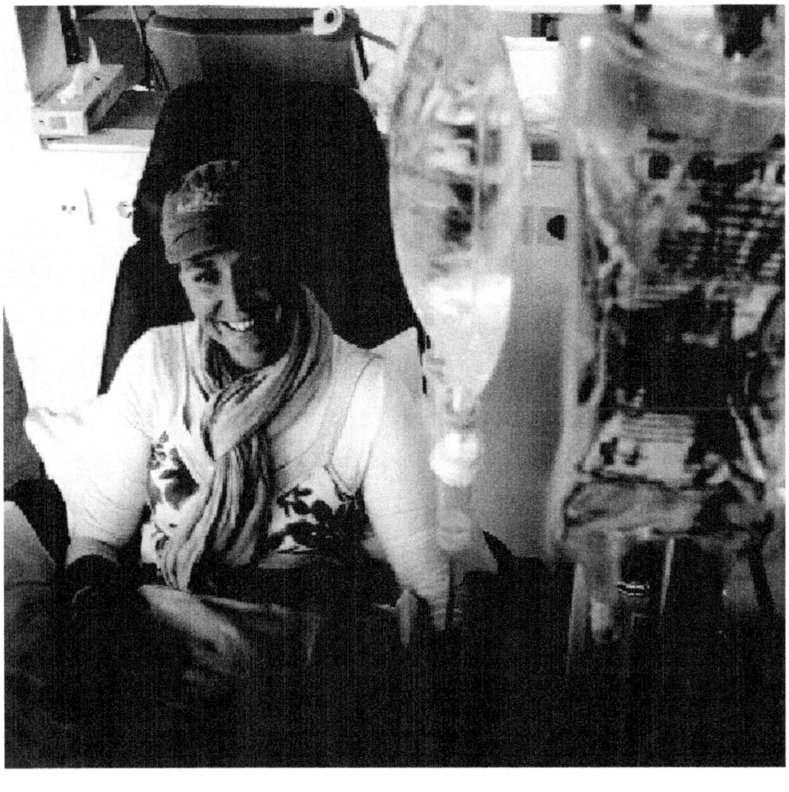

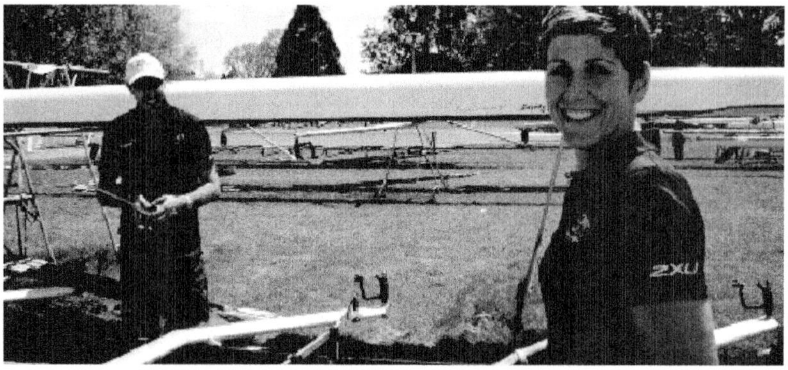

"Coming from a sports background, it helped me to visualise the whole treatment as my "race for the cure". A triathlon with the three disciplines – chemo, surgery and radiation. I had to make it through all three individually, step by step, kilometre by kilometre, and every discipline was a challenge in itself."

If I had done a self-examination of the breast, or even just paid more attention when I was putting on body lotion, I would have been able to feel the tumour sooner and probably would have noticed before it reached grade three and had spread to my lymph nodes."Getting fit again after treatment has been a challenge and a long journey. At the same time it's been great to see how your body can recover."

"Of course cancer can strike randomly, but you have to control the things you can control – stay out of the sun, don't smoke, exercise regularly, eat fruit and vegetables. By doing these things,

you're already reducing your risk by a large percentage."

"I experienced a lot of strength in the people around me. Unfortunately I also experienced a lot of ignorance, apprehension and insecurity in how to deal with me. I now understand that some of the reactions were just peoples' fear of their own mortality. It was not actually about me, my bald head or my grey face."

In 2008, Cora Zillich, age 41, noticed a swelling in her left armpit, which she thought may have been an infected sweat gland. She was sent for an ultrasound and a 3 cm tumour, which had already begun to spread to her lymph nodes, was found in her left breast. Being told she had cancer was already shocking, but when they threw in the words 'aggressive', 'advanced' and 'fast growing', it was pretty hard to deal with. Cora made it her mission to find out as much as possible about cancer, and cancer treatment, and to educate as many people as she could. She is currently in remission.

"I now say, "A bad day in any normal situation is still better than any day in cancer treatment."

ANDRE VINCENT

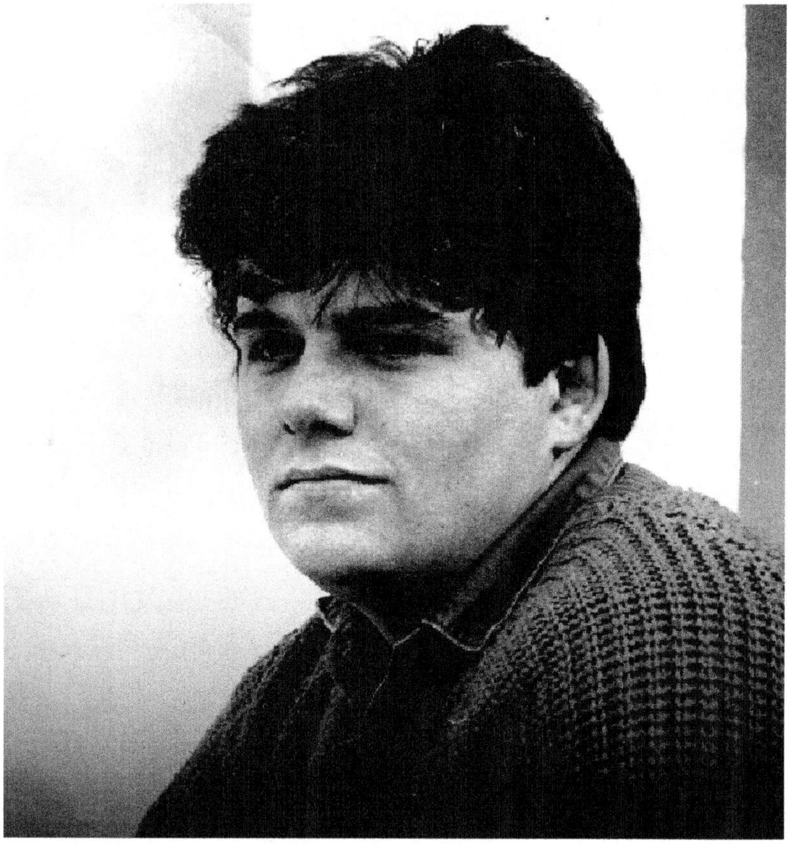

A lot of people still have that British "stiff upper lip" Victorian values way of dealing with cancer. "It will never find us if we never speak its name." It's amazing how much negativity you get from people who can't even say the word. It's always "illness", "health scare", or "little issue". Some people even said, "You should not talk about it so freely, and you certainly should not do jokes about it."

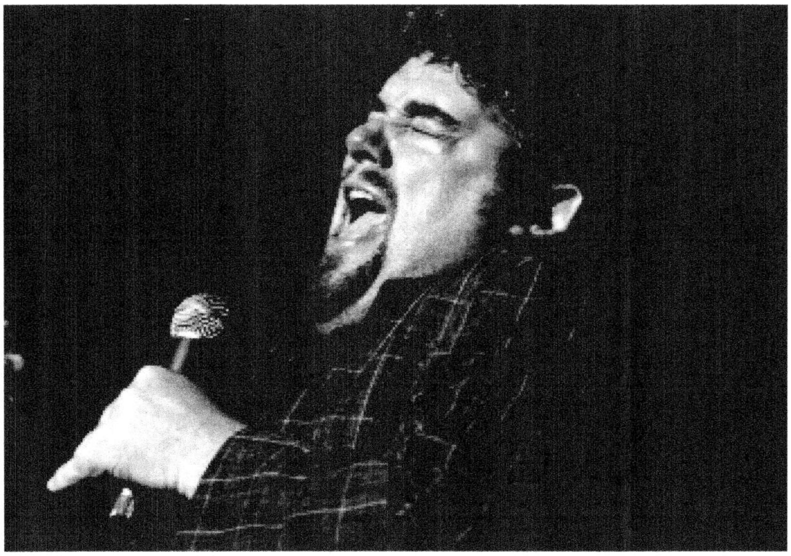

The day English stand up comic, Andre Vincent, 46, was diagnosed with cancer he thought he wouldn't tell anyone and would just get on with life. Three of his comedy heroes Andy Kaufman, Graham Chapman and Bill Hicks had all died of cancer and not one of them told an audience, so he thought he'd be the same. That night he had a gig and during it someone heckled him. André heard himself say 'No, don't – I got cancer' and then told the audience the news he had received earlier that day. Then, to a slightly confused and muted crowd, he brought on the next act, fellow comic George Egg. To this day George still reminds André of the long, silent walk he had to the microphone. André went on to turn his experiences into an award winning one man show called 'Hoorah for Cancer', which he performed at the Edinburgh Fringe Festival to enormous acclaim.

"Hey, it's my cancer, I'll do what I please with it."

"People would tell me I had a great way of dealing with cancer, but you don't deal with your cancer, most of the time you're dealing with everyone else dealing with your cancer."

When he was in for treatment, the hospital insisted he wear pyjamas – but he didn't own a pair. His girlfriend found some South Park material and made him some PJ's, which meant there was a big fat child running loose around the hospital wards.

"I never get down or depressed, I never let things get on top of me. There is the old adage, "If life gives you lemons, make lemonade." I've now added to that "And learn how to package it and sell it".

"When a counsellor gives you their very best "empathy" face, pats your hand gently and says, "Remember, cancer is a word, not a sentence" she doesn't want to hear, "It's also a star sign, ***and*** **one of the tropics!"**

MARTIN MASON

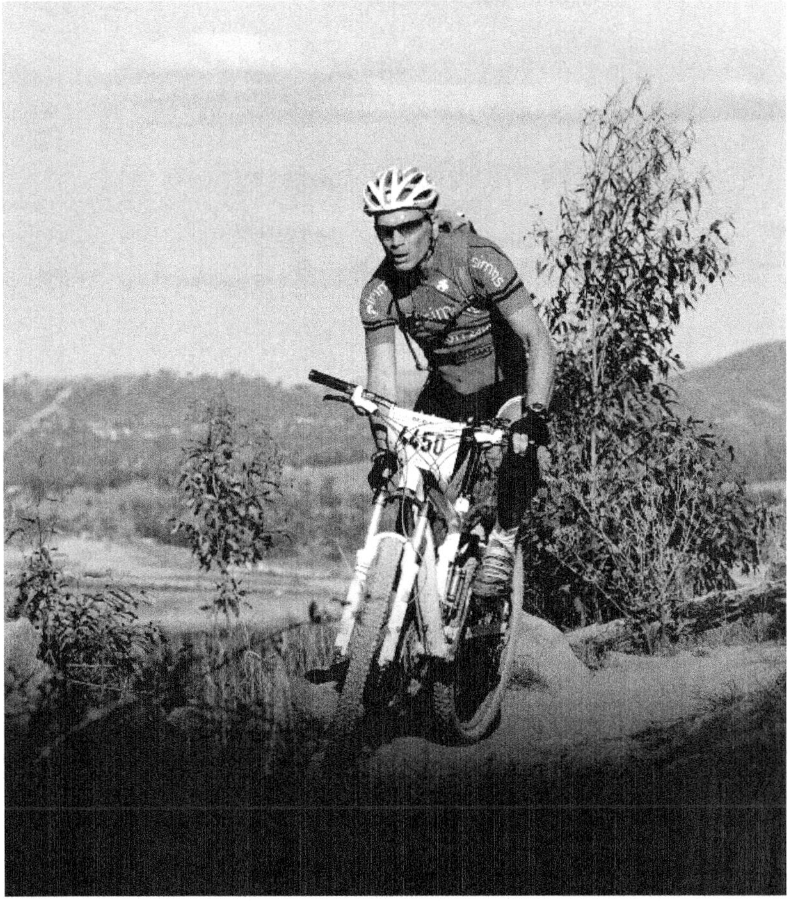

"I guess everybody would feel – like I did initially – that "having cancer" is almost a death sentence. The reality is that it's not. There's certainly some share of cancers, like testicular cancer, that are very curable: 99 percent curable."

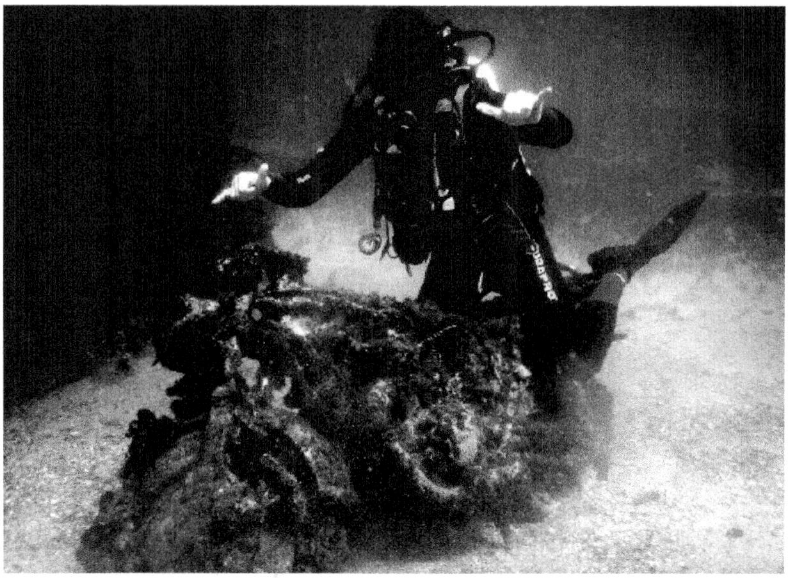

"Talking about "your bits" is embarrassing and the last thing you want to do is show them to anybody. It's almost a taboo subject, but if you have *any* doubt about *anything* at all, you have to go and see your GP and they can usually tell very quickly."

When he was 46, Martin Mason casually mentioned to his wife, Kathy, that he'd had a recurring pain in his testicle for some time. Kathy got straight onto the phone and booked Martin in for an appointment with his GP. He was immediately sent for an ultrasound, and later that day was told the words no one ever wants to hear, 'You have cancer.' Martin was quickly referred to a specialist and was assured that testicular cancer is very curable. Even though this was years ago, and Martin has made a complete recovery, to this day, whenever Martin thinks about hearing those words, it gives him shivers.

"Cancer has had an enormously positive effect on my life. I think I'm a nicer person, I'm in touch with my emotions and it's brought me much closer to my family."

WARRICK TRY

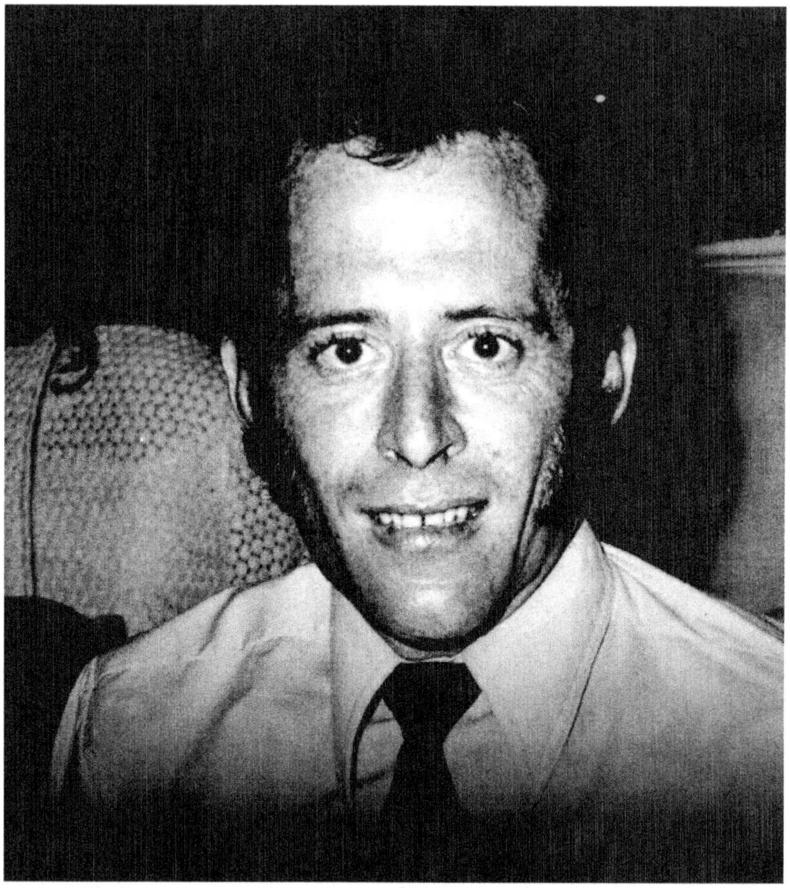

"Be very careful with your health, fitness and lifestyle. Don't do anything too excessive because in the end your bad habits will win. I didn't get married until I was 35 so around 30 I was young, single, plenty of money and doing ridiculous things to my body. And whilst it's very difficult to make a young person listen, I think you have to have to try and say to them "Don't do this to your body. It will catch up to you."

Warrick Try, 68, partied pretty hard into his thirties and smoked until he was 50. Then, six years after quitting cigarettes, he started feeling a little breathless but put it down to old age creeping up. Then some x-rays after a skiing accident revealed he had cancer which had almost closed off his right lung. At the time Warrick had a wife and five children, the youngest being only five. He had an operation to remove his lung, and this was hoped to have gotten rid of the cancer. Since then, Warrick has cancer of the bladder, the prostate, the eye and several malignant melanomas.

"When cancer is first diagnosed, some people start to die almost immediately, others start to live. The choice is yours."

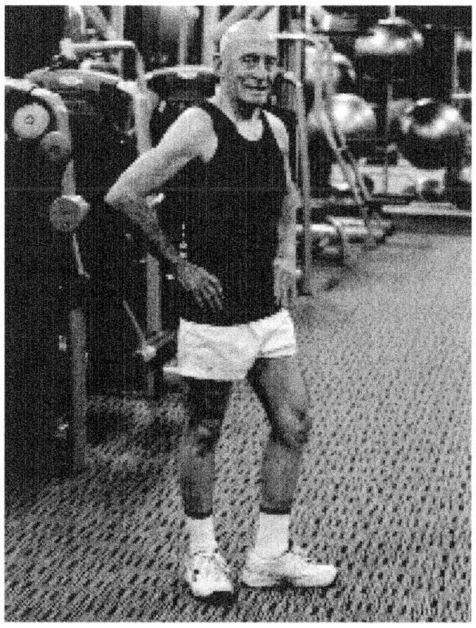

In December 2009 it was discovered that his PSA levels had risen – his prostate cancer was back – and a course of chemotherapy was recommended. Warrick decided to get his body as fit as possible to help his chances of getting through the chemo well. He went to the gym, changed his diet, and improved his whole lifestyle. In an amazing turnaround, Warrick quickly saw dramatic changes in his body shape and fitness, and his PSA levels got lower and lower. In his latest blood test it's down to 0.001 – almost undetectable – and for the first time in twelve years the doctors have pronounced Warrick cancer free.

"You can defeat cancer, it's not all-powerful, lots of people overcome it. A positive attitude won't definitely beat cancer, but laying down and getting all depressed will definitely promote it."

URSULA HARVEY

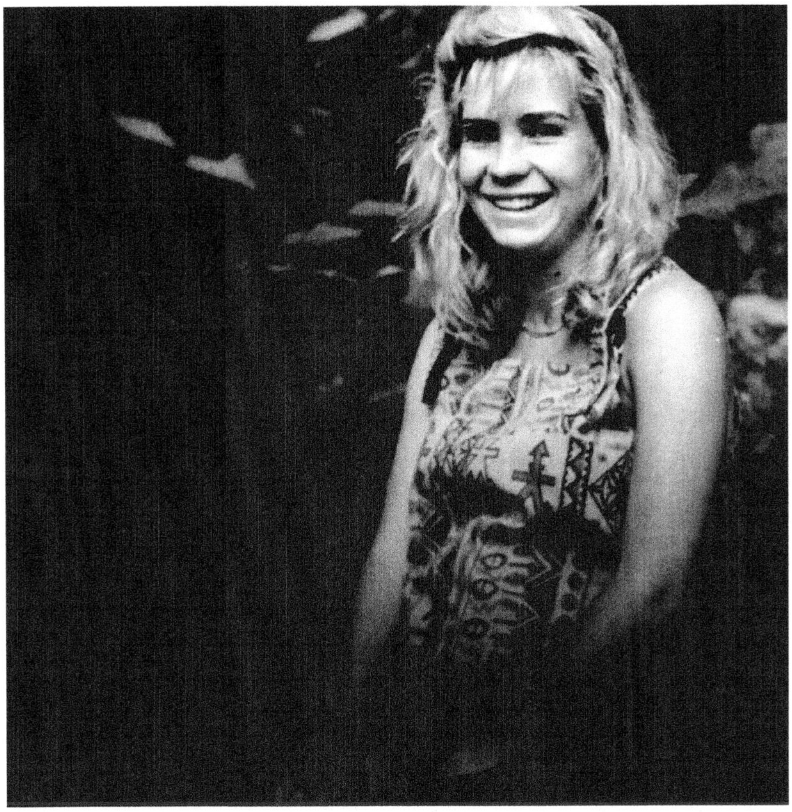

"I wish I knew that it is NORMAL to be scared!"

"I wish that other people knew it was okay to laugh with you when you have cancer."

"I wish people knew that when you have fought a really good fight and have lost, that it is okay. You did your best! It is up to them now to continue the fight when you are gone."

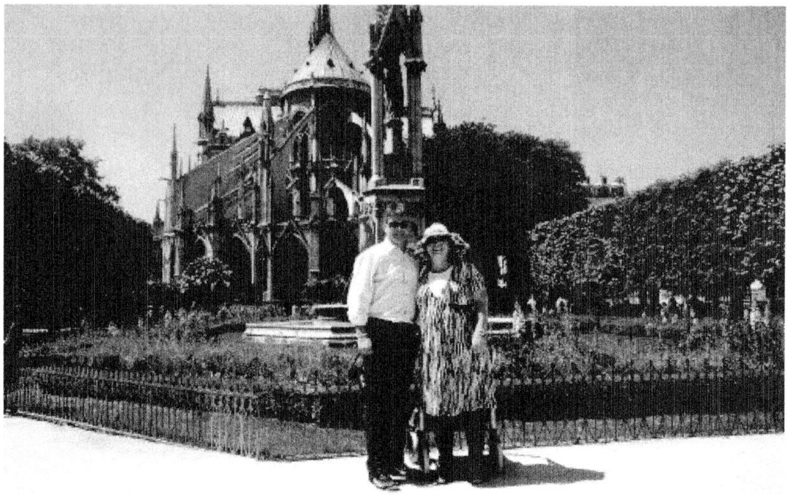

In May, 2010, Ursula Harvey and her hubby celebrated one year 'still being here' after diagnosis. They went to France, had lunch in the Eiffel Tower did a 'toast to life'.

"I wish I knew how to tell people that it is HARD when they tell you to "stay positive." That same person will probably go home and cry because I have cancer. But I have to "stay positive". Give me a friend who will cry with me, and then help me fight.""I wish I knew how much it would hurt when people I loved and cared about dropped out of my life when I was diagnosed. I guess they figured I had reached my use-by date."

"I wish I had known what a blessing it was going to be in the long run, few people get to find out who their true friends are but I did and they will be treasured in my heart always."

"I wish people knew that listening is the best gift you can give someone with cancer. Listen to them talk, listen to the hurt, listen to the silence, just be there and listen."

"I wish I had known how precious my life is to me!"

"I wish I knew if I will get the chance to see my children graduate or play with my grandchildren one day."

DALE CLIFF

"Continue to believe. Be incredibly positive. Irrespective of what the diagnosis might be, be positive. The minute you stop believing, is the minute it will end on you."

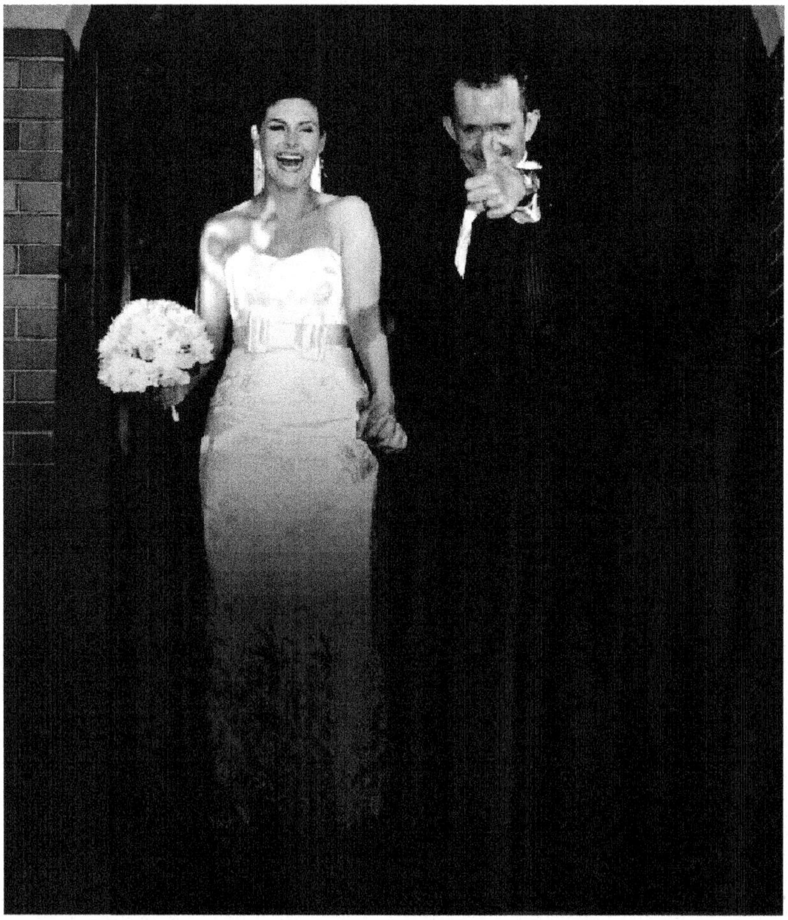

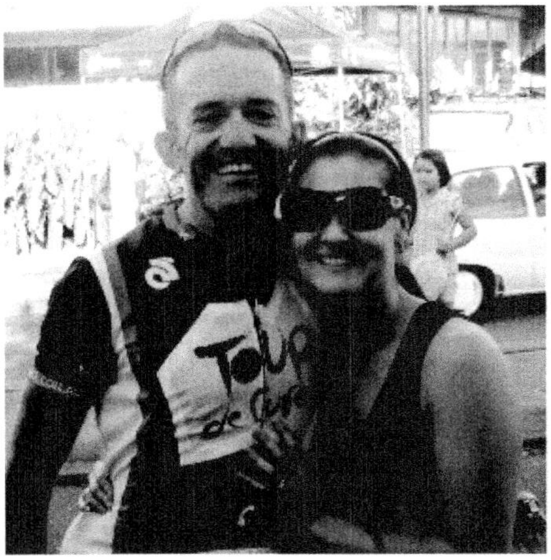

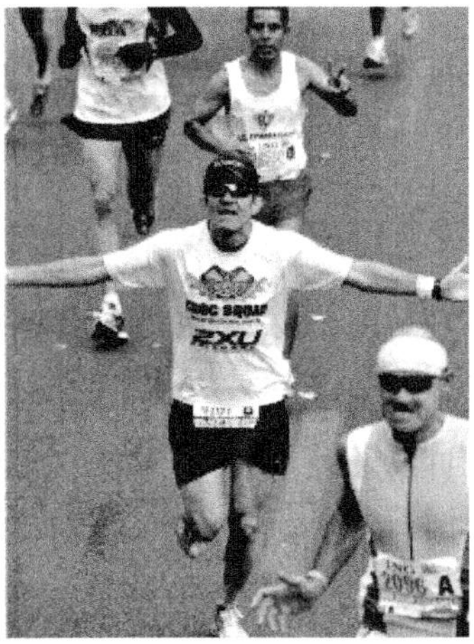

"You just have to keep moving forward. If you look back in life, you get a sore neck."

In 2005, after just having finished the Hawaiian Ironman competition, Dale, now aged 45, noticed his health deteriorating. In 2006, his speech started to disappear and his thought patterns became interrupted. He put it down to stress. In late 2006, at the insistence of his colleagues, he went and saw a GP and was sent for a CT scan. Dale was told he had a brain tumour and had 6–12 months to live. He went in for surgery the following week and it was found that, miraculously, the tumour had not penetrated his brain and was able to be taken out without any need for chemotherapy or radiation. Dale now lives with the knowledge that there is a 75 percent chance the tumour will grow back.

"There are some people in your life who become so much more important in the darkness after

diagnosis. People who have always been around, but they suddenly take a front seat in your life."

Cancer taught me that you only have so many weekends left in your life: you can literally count them. I abjectly refuse to work weekends now because I want to make the most of this time. "Ironically, getting life back to normal is a hard thing for cancer survivors. There's the initial trauma we all go through, and then there's the ongoing recovery. By that time your friends and family have had to move on and get back to their own lives."

EPILOGUE

What started as an idea over coffee between two mates has quickly become Australia's leading cycling foundation and along the way helps spread the message of research, support and prevention of cancer. The Tour de Cure has raised millions of dollars in the fight against cancer for men, women and children. The Tour de Cure is a cycling foundation that brings together ordinary people to take on extraordinary events to shorten the distance of curing cancer. Every member of the Tour de Cure team dreams of the day when front page headlines read of a cure being found. Until that time, the crew, riders and ambassadors who are part of the Tour de Cure tribe hope to spread the message of what can be done to lessen the chances of men, women and children having to face cancer. The Tour hopes to provide support to those people living with cancer and fund much needed research in order to find a cure.

To find out how to be a part of the Tour de Cure visit www.tourdecure.com.au.

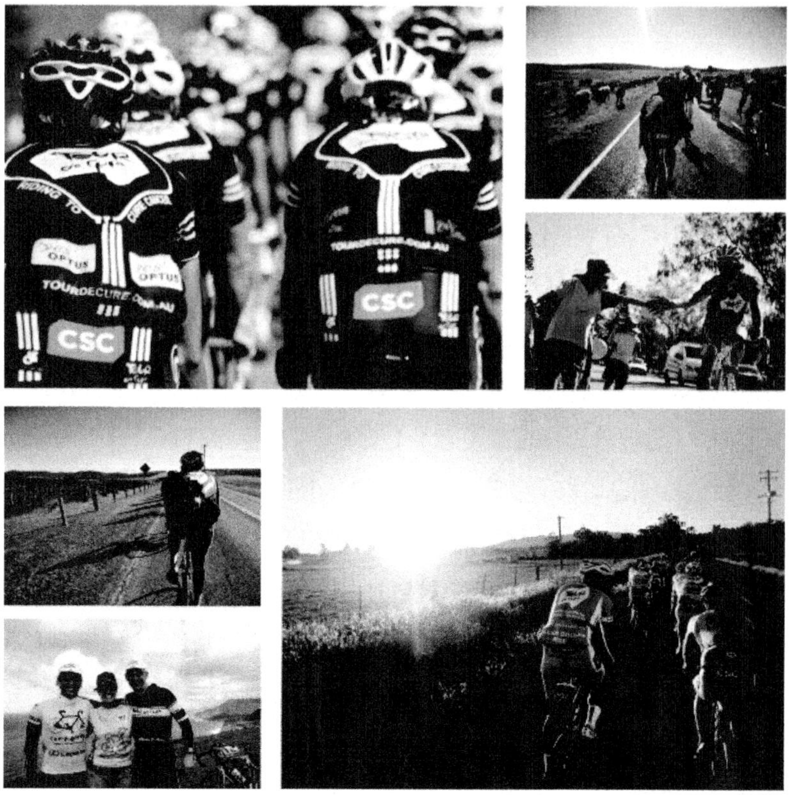

Pfizer Oncology

Pfizer Oncology is committed to the discovery, investigation and development of innovative treatment options to improve the outlook for cancer patients worldwide. As science in oncology continues to evolve, Pfizer is pursuing research centred around a personalised approach to cancer treatment and tailoring therapy based on the molecular and/or biologic make-up of the disease. Our robust pipeline consists of 22 biologics and small molecules in development, including several first-in-class compounds.

We are currently running over 200 clinical trials, including 14 phase III trials, in some of the most prevalent and difficult-to-treat cancers such as lung, prostate, colorectal, breast, liver, and renal cell. Our goal is to provide patients with better, more customised treatment options with longer survival rates in various tumour types.

Pfizer Oncology works collaboratively with academic institutions, individual researchers, cooperative research groups, governments and licensing partners to further its extensive research and development program. We are committed to partnerships with professional and patient organisations that deliver benefits to patients including disease management tools, awareness of clinical trial options and access to new medicines.

Working together, we strive to transform treatment by targeting the right drug for the right patient at the right time.

Pfizer Oncology understands that helping people with cancer goes beyond medicines and, by partnering with like minded organisations who share the same vision to help people with cancer, we can achieve a lot more than we can working alone. Through our partnership with Tour de Cure we hope to provide support to patients and their carers, further research in cancer treatment and help prevent cancer through raising awareness and education.

Pfizer Oncology is proud to be a Platinum Sponsor of Tour de Cure.

G.J. Gardner. HOMES

Curing cancer is possible. I know that now because my father is a cancer survivor. When Dad was diagnosed with non-Hodgkin's cancer five years ago, I was optimistic and a little arrogant. I thought to myself, 'these days cancer can be cured'. I assumed someone somewhere was doing the hard yards to cure cancer and I left them to it. Dad did beat cancer and is now fitter than ever. He gets his regular check-ups and likes to tell us all how he passes with flying colours. Maybe this disease won't affect me again on a personal level, but one thing is for sure, my thoughts about cancer have changed. Curing cancer is possible. I know that now because my father is a cancer survivor. When Dad was diagnosed with non-Hodgkin's cancer five years ago, I was optimistic and a little arrogant. I thought to myself, 'these days cancer can be cured'. I assumed someone somewhere was doing the hard yards to cure cancer and I left them to it. Dad did beat cancer and is now fitter than ever. He gets his regular check-ups and likes to tell us all how he passes with flying colours. Maybe this disease won't affect me again on a personal level, but one thing is for sure, my thoughts about cancer have changed.

Before my father's diagnosis, cancer was a disease someone else had with a cure someone else was researching. After hearing Dad's stories of other cancer patients who didn't survive, I realised that not all families are as lucky as ours. When I met Gary Bertwistle, the co-founder of Tour de Cure, his drive and passion for helping raise money to find a cure for cancer was truly inspirational.

The more I got to know about Gary, and the work he was doing with Tour de Cure, the more I discovered that with my strong business contacts and a network of friends I really could make a difference and at the same time give back to those people who helped save my Dad.

Working for G.J. Gardner Homes, a franchise building company, provided the perfect platform to get involved. G.J. Gardner homes is extremely strong and passionate about everything we do, and supporting the community. Choosing Tour de Cure as our charity has generated over-whelming interest and support from our franchisees, employees, suppliers and sub-contractors.

As a large organisation we are proud to have been able to raise awareness and money across Australia for research into a cure for cancer-and it's only the beginning. Many fund-raising events are on the horizon aimed at getting whole communities involved in a range of activities from town biking events to raffles and much more. Our ultimate goal is to build a comfortable home for cancer patients to stay in while they undergo treatment for cancer.

G.J. Gardner Homes feel passionate about the research, support and prevention of cancer. We are proud to support Tour de Cure and excited to be a part of this book of invaluable information.

From the team at G.J. Gardner Homes, we wish the riders the very best on the tour and encourage you to donate to the Tour de Cure.

Jarrod Blamey

ACKNOWLEDGMENTS

Marty and Gary would like to thank all those people who generously shared their stories to make the lives of others better. And a special and enormous thanks goes to our publisher Denny Neave from Big Sky Publishing, you are a rock. Thanks mate.

Marty also thanks Gary Bertwistle. You gotta love people who make stuff happen. Tour de Cure. Ditto. Dan Gregory for cranking WIWIK up with me. Mathew Alderson for the occasional 'Whoah there, big fella.' My wife, Allie. Together we make a great team: She is brilliant, patient, resilient and supportive. I am grateful. My two boys, Connor and Elliot, for understanding that Dadda brought his 'stupid laptop' on our holiday to get this book done.

Gary would also like to thank the passion behind the Tour de Cure, cofounder Geoff "Cougar" Coombes, the engine behind the tour, Samantha Hollier-James, and the brains behind the tour, Bruno Maurel plus the energy of our board from Dom and Julie. Thanks Gabbi for making my words make sense, Jake and Vienda for being my backbone. I appreciate it.

Printed in Dunstable, United Kingdom

91220109R00078